ONE DOCTOR:

A PHYSICIAN'S DIARY

ONE DOCTOR:

A PHYSICIAN'S DIARY

Thomas Marzili, M.D.

To order additional copies of this book, contact:
Xlibris Corporation
1-888-795-4274
www.Xlibris.com
Orders@Xlibris.com
29577

Contents

To my wife, Laurie
My toughest critic and most loving supporter

Introduction

"What do you do for a living?"

This question arises in the course of almost every conversation with a new acquaintance. There are many answers that garner but a nod of acknowledgement and then on to the next question. My answer to that question is that "I am a doctor." From that point on, the conversation becomes easy. People always have medical questions or seize the opportunity for free medical advice. But more often they want to hear the stories of the people and the cases that make the medical profession so fascinating.

Since I was a small child I had wanted to be a doctor. Like most children, I did not know what an accountant, an engineer, a banker or a systems analyst really did. But like all children, I knew what a doctor did. I had always dreamed of becoming a doctor but as I began my final year in high school I had made no definite plans.

That changed on an early October day in 1979 as I sat in the third floor classroom of Haddon Heights High School and stared out the window at an unusual early autumn snowfall. My teacher was teaching Physics but my mind was a million miles away. Prior to that day, I had been investigating colleges and plotting my career course without any true direction. But on that day, October 10, 1979, I received my calling.

I have heard priests and nuns talk about getting a calling but never fully understood what they meant. Perhaps I was even skeptical that such a thing existed. But as I looked out into the snow on that remarkable October day, the desire to become a doctor permeated my mind and my heart and was so overwhelming that I knew it could never be denied.

I wish I could say that my road to medicine was a straight and unobstructed course, but there were doubts and detours along the way. Yet there were always influential people and circumstances that came at the right times in my life to help set me back along my path.

On a breezy, cool day in May of 1990, I achieved my dream and received my medical degree. It was not the completion of a dream but only the beginning.

The next three years were spent in residency and I have been practicing medicine ever since. On a busy day now I may see fifty or sixty patients. But I always remember that each patient is seeing but one doctor. Every encounter is important and memorable. There is nothing more rewarding than helping a person at a critical point in their life. Nearly everyone can remember a time when they were deathly ill, frightened, depressed or hopeless and turned to a doctor for help.

The impact of a doctor's care to his patients will outlast his career and his memories will outlast his life. I consider myself so very fortunate to have the opportunity to work in what I consider the greatest profession in the world. To be afforded the chance to share and influence my patients' lives in such a positive way.

What do I do for a living?

Talk to any doctor and he could spend hours talking about fascinating cases and people that he has encountered throughout his career. But these are just my stories. And I am just one doctor.

1

The Beginning

Day One

I sat up anxiously from my bed and turned down the call room TV as I nervously fumbled for my beeper. It was the first day of my residency, my first day as a doctor.

I placed a clipboard full of notes on my lap, pulled a Merck manual and Physicians' Desk Reference close to me on the bed and felt sorry for the poor souls who found themselves in the hospital during the first week of July. My white coat dangled from a coat hook on the door. On the left chest was my name followed by the letters M.D. At home I had a diploma that also identified me as a medical doctor. But I was not yet a doctor. A doctor would not be sitting in a cold sweat every time the pager went off.

I quickly dialed the number and identified myself.

"A patient needs to be pronounced in 642," the nurse calmly stated.

My immediate reaction was one of relief. I paged through my clipboard that contained tips on how to handle several emergencies. Chest pain, shortness of breath, change in mental status. It sounds horrible to say now, but at the time I was glad that he did not have any of those more difficult problems where my skills would be put to the test. I was relieved that he was only dead. I quickly located the instructions on completing a death certificate and made my way to his room.

As I arrived at the nurses' station, the secretary handed me the patient's chart and pointed me towards his room. I quickly glanced through his chart. He was a seventy-nine year old man with lung cancer that had spread to his bones and brain. There was a "Do Not Resuscitate" order and the last few physician notes indicated that death was imminent.

I walked down the hall and nervously entered his dimly lit room. I expected to find his nurse or a family member but there was no one. I slowly approached his bed. He was skin and bones. His skin was ghostly white and his eyes were sunken but open. His toothless mouth was wide open and his lips were parched.

I pulled a flashlight from my pocket and shined it into his eyes. His pupils were fixed and dilated. I took my stethoscope and gently pressed it against his chest. I moved it around to several spots over his heart. Nothing. As I removed my stethoscope, I fumbled with it and dropped it onto his chest.

"I'm sorry," I reflexively said then looked around to see if anyone had seen me.

I sat down in the chair next to his bed to complete the paperwork. Suddenly I was struck by the fact that I was sitting alone in a dark room with a dead body. It was a situation that I would eventually get used to, but that was my first time and it was rather spooky. It was the first time I was frightened as a doctor. I would be frightened plenty of more times in the future, but never again in that way.

I tried to shrug it off and turned my attention to the death certificate. I filled out the cause of death: Lung cancer. He was dead to God and dead to the world but his death was not official in the eyes of the state until I completed his death certificate. It gives one a strange sense of power though I knew it was just a formality.

I carefully wrote his name. I signed my name at the bottom, then added M.D. with a flourish. I wrote the time: 10:42 PM. I paused before writing the date. I looked back at his lifeless body and suddenly felt an ironic bond with this man whom I had never known.

I finally etched the date: July 1, 1990. His family would forever sadly remember it as the last day of his life, the date of his death. But despite my fears and uncertainty, I will always treasure it as my first day as a doctor.

2

Medical School

First Patient

She would be the first patient we would see during our medical school careers. There was excitement in the air as we crowded into the physical therapy room in anticipation of her arrival. It was the second semester of my first year in medical school and we were visiting a rehabilitation center for patients who had suffered neurological injuries.

Up until that time, medical school had been textbooks, lecture halls, and laboratories. It would be our first chance to see the practical application of our studies in actual patients. It was a welcome change of scenery.

"Good morning, everyone," the neurologist proudly said, "we have a few very interesting neurological cases who have volunteered to help in your education."

We all sat wide-eyed in anticipation as the first patient was wheeled in. She was a beautiful young girl, about seventeen years old, with long blonde hair pulled back in a ponytail. She was a thin, athletic looking girl who appeared nervous as she entered.

"Our first case," he began, casting a brief glance in her direction, "has been with us a short time. About a month ago she was in a motor vehicle accident, suffered a cervical fracture and severely damaged her spinal cord. The driver was killed. She was actually very lucky."

I did not know much about neurology, but from where I was sitting she did not look very lucky. Her body may have been paralyzed by the accident but her face looked paralyzed by fear. Her eyes wandered the room but she avoided eye contact with any of us. I thought she was going to cry but she bravely did not.

The neurologist walked over to her, lifted her arm from the wheelchair, released it and let it fall back to the arm rest.

"Dead weight," he proudly stated, then looking at her he loudly ordered, "Okay, now try to hold your arm up."

Again he demonstratively lifted her arm, released it, and let it fall helplessly down.

"Nothing," he hollered as tears welled in the girl's terrified eyes.

He then grasped her wrist and lifted her hand.

"Move your fingers," he commanded. I did not see any movement.

"Did you see that?" He excitedly said. "Did you see that? Now, can anyone tell me at which level her spinal cord is severed?"

The hands went up on a few eager students while the rest of us sat there with our mouths open in horror at the spectacle that we were witnessing.

Undoubtedly, the young woman had interesting neurological deficits that could help reinforce the neuroanatomy we were learning in the classroom. But as I looked at that interesting medical case I saw only a young girl who would never go dancing with her friends, would never take a walk along the beach or down the aisle at her wedding. I saw a girl who would forever be confined to a wheelchair and dependent on others for the basic necessities of life.

The neurologist was in his glory in front of the audience and totally oblivious to the young girl's feeling. As I watched my first patient, I wondered how many years and how many patients it would take before I could look at a patient and no longer see a person. I wondered how long it would take until I viewed a patient as only a medical case consisting of signs, symptoms and test results. I looked at the stunned faces of most of my fellow students. I wondered. I hoped. I hoped never.

Four Dollars

I took a deep breath and composed myself before entering the hospital room. I was a third year medical student and preparing myself to deliver bad news. I was well aware that I had never done this before. He had a resident, an attending physician, and a lung specialist all caring for him, but I was the one who saw him three or four times a day. I was the one who spent the most time with him and I felt that I should deliver the news.

He had entered the hospital three days earlier after several days of coughing and more recently coughing up blood. He was a fifty-eight year old sometimes laborer. He was an indigent patient with no insurance. He had an address, but he had lived on and off the streets.

"Good afternoon," I nervously said as I entered the room although I knew it wasn't going to be a good afternoon.

He sat in a chair beside the bed staring at a blank TV screen. "Afternoon," he said with a nod in my direction.

"Are you watching TV?" I asked.

"Naw, man," he said with a chuckle, "cost four dollar for the TV. I ain't got no four dollar."

"How about something to read," I suggested, "there's plenty of magazines in the lounge."

"Ain't never learned to read," he answered. He did not seem insulted but I felt bad for having suggested it. I should have realized he was illiterate but at the time I had never met someone who could not read.

"Anyway, I came to talk to you about your bronchoscopy results," I said, "the biopsies finally came back."

"Cancer?" he asked, taking me aback.

"Uh, I'm afraid so," I nervously replied, "but we're going to take care of you. You're going to be evaluated further tomorrow so we can come up with a treatment plan."

"Pretty bad, huh," he said, "my daddy died of the cancer."

"I'm sorry," I said. "Do you have any family to be with you tonight?"

"Naw," he said sadly, "got three kids I ain't seen in years. I've been trying to reach my sister but she don't know I'm here."

He continued to stare at the blank TV screen. He had a hopeless look and tears welled in his eyes.

I stood there as an inexperienced, naive third year medical student. I did not know much about doctor-patient relationships, boundaries or proper protocol. I struggled for the right words but the room remained silent. I reached into my wallet and pulled out four dollars and laid it on his bed.

"Here," I said, "I'll get the lady to come back and turn on your TV."

"Thank you," he said with a surprised but ecstatic look.

I looked in on him before I left for the night and he was smiling and staring intently at the TV. For that moment, his troubles were forgotten.

I knew that what I did for him would not make any major difference in the overall scheme of things, but I will never forget the look on his face that night. And when I look back, I have no doubt that it was the best four dollars I had ever spent.

Homeless and Pregnant

I pulled my lab coat tightly against the freezing February air as it whipped through the Emergency Department every time the door opened and closed for another unfortunate patient. I was doing my Emergency Medicine rotation as part of my fourth year of medical school and was amazed at how many patients braved the winter chill to seek medical care.

I glanced at the presenting complaint of my first patient. She was a twenty-three year old woman who had come in with contractions although she was only five months pregnant. Her address was a homeless shelter. She was lying on a stretcher as I entered the room, her boyfriend standing protectively by her side. I asked her what had brought her in.

"She's having contractions," her boyfriend answered, "she needs to be in a hospital. We're really worried about the baby."

"How often are they coming?" I asked.

"On and off," her boyfriend answered, "but they're real strong. We need to keep an eye on her."

The young woman nodded softly in agreement.

I asked her a few more questions and examined her, then arranged for her to go to Labor and Delivery to be monitored. As a lowly medical student, I also had the honor of transporting her. I helped her into the wheelchair and we made our way down the hall.

"I'm staying with her," her boyfriend said as I wheeled her down the quiet corridor, "it's my baby too. I'll just sleep in a recliner. They let me do it last time."

He seemed excited to sleep in a recliner. I had slept in one myself and they were far from comfortable. But I was comparing it to a mattress and comforter and not cement and cardboard.

I waited as the nurse placed a monitor on the patient. I was still too inexperienced to realize what was going on.

"Will she need to be admitted?" I asked.

The nurse smiled pleasantly at the patient then led me out of the room.

"She's no more in labor than you are," she said with a roll of her eyes. "This is the third time she's been here. They're just looking for a warm room for the night. A few more minutes on the monitor and they're out of here. I feel bad for them. But we're busy. We're not a homeless shelter."

I stood there silently as the nurse broke the news to the dejected couple. I then faced the unpleasant task of escorting them back to the emergency room.

"This is ridiculous," her boyfriend shouted as we waited for the elevator, "how could they not give her a room? What if she has her baby on the street? I can't believe this hospital. We have good insurance."

"You have insurance?" I asked, immediately regretting the surprise in my voice.

"We have Medicaid," he proudly answered.

I wheeled her back to her room and told her to take off her gown and put on her street clothes. The words "street clothes" sounded as though I was describing some sort of uniform for street people and I felt bad for saying it. Apologizing would have only made matters worse.

I filled out their discharge forms and had the young woman sign them. I handed them back their copy, which the young man angrily crumbled and threw into the trashcan. I knew that the nurse in Labor and Delivery had done the right thing. The hospital had saved countless hours of work and expensive testing that were medically unnecessary. The state Medicaid insurance had saved several hundred and perhaps thousands of dollars in pointless medical expenses. But that was little consolation for a fourth year medical student as I pulled my collar tightly around my neck and turned my back on a pregnant woman as she walked out onto the icy streets on a frigid February evening.

Pieta

Pieta. It is one of Michelangelo's most magnificent sculptures depicting the Virgin Mary holding the lifeless body of her son Jesus Christ after his crucifixion. Jesus looks so peaceful in his Mother's arms as Mary looks mournfully down at her Son. It is the portrayal of the most sorrowful event of Christianity yet I am amazed at the shear beauty of the sculpture.

I could have seen *Pieta.* I could have gone to Rome and seen St. Peter's Basilica. But I was a struggling medical student and such an extravagant Spring Break during my fourth year of school was far beyond my means. So on that spring day in my final year of medical school I found myself riding through the streets of North Camden with a hospice nurse to visit a dying patient.

We pulled up to a dingy row home in a squalid neighborhood. Two of the first floor windows were boarded up and trash was strewn on the porch. The nurse gathered some equipment and got out of the car. I followed her closely as we passed a small group of young men standing aimlessly on the sidewalk. I feared for my life and wondered if the car would still be there when we returned. She smiled at one of the men and he nodded slightly in recognition.

We knocked at the door and a woman answered and warmly welcomed the nurse. The nurse introduced me and the woman graciously shook my hand. The woman appeared to be about sixty years old and the victim of a hard life. Her gray hair was straggly and thinning. Most of her teeth were missing and her face bore a deep scar across her left cheek. But she was not the patient.

She led us upstairs to a depressing little room where her twenty-eight year old son lay dying of AIDS. It was an old house and the room appeared filthy. The furniture was old and broken, the walls looked like they had not been painted in fifty years, and there were magazines and newspapers scattered on the floor that looked like they had been there for months.

The young man was nothing but skin and bones. He could not have weighed more than sixty pounds. He was naked but for a dirty sheet that was pulled to his waist. His hair was long, uncombed and unclean. He appeared to have not been shaven in weeks and had a beard that contained particles of food and dried blood.

A stench filled the room. I felt pity for the young man but felt only repulsion for the scene. I wanted the visit to end so we could leave as soon as possible.

I stood by, careful not to lean on anything, as the nurse asked the mother several questions about the young man's progress. I was impressed by the mother's answers. Despite the conditions in which they lived, she seemed to be taking loving and meticulous care of her son. But there was a painful strain in her voice. She was doing everything she could for him yet she knew she could not prevent his death.

We examined the young man. He barely responded to our questions. He seemed to be in pain, agitated and suffering greatly. We tried to lift him to examine a bedsore but he resisted our movement. We then tried to roll him over but were again unsuccessful.

"You wanna look at his back?" his mother asked.

We nodded.

She sat down on his bed and softly whispered into his ear. She then placed her arms underneath him and lifted him up like a baby onto her lap. His head fell back but she caught it and held it in her arms. His long, thin arms and legs dangled from under the sheet that was draped over him. He no longer appeared to be in pain but seemed to be at peace. His mother looked down upon him with the most sorrowful yet beautiful expression. Amid the deplorable conditions in that room on that day, I was deeply touched by the beauty of the long suffering mother's undying love for her dying son that she cradled tenderly in her arms. There was a beauty in her sorrow that was beyond what mere words could describe, a beauty that could only be captured by the likes of Michelangelo.

I never made it to Rome. I never visited the Basilica of St. Peter. But on that April day in North Camden, I had found *Pieta*.

Judgment Day

"Are you remembering to give her the antibiotic," he asked in a stern but caring manner.

"Sure," she casually answered, "I might forget from time to time but usually I remember."

The pediatrician studied the mother thoughtfully. He was a diminutive man with a bookish face and a timid manner. It may not have been clear to me as a third year medical student but it was obvious to this seasoned physician that the little girl was not getting her medication.

"Have a seat on the table," he said in a friendly reassuring way to the four year old girl as she hopped onto the examining table. He joked playfully with the delightful little girl as he methodically examined her from head to toe.

The girl looked fairly healthy except for being small for her age and for the noticeably swollen lymph nodes in her neck.

"She looks great," he said to me with a smile, "but you should have seen her in the hospital. She was a sick little girl. Her neck was three times this size. You can look at the chart."

I began perusing the chart and quickly realized that the little girl was much sicker than I had first recognized. The child was born to an HIV infected mother and at her tender age already had AIDS. She had a two year old sister who was also infected. The mother, although HIV positive for years, had shown no overt signs of AIDS. It was 1988 and the treatments for HIV paled in comparison to the treatments of today.

I glanced at the mother. She was an attractive young Hispanic woman dressed in jeans and a maternity shirt. I wondered how a young woman who was already sending two children to an early death could bring another baby into the world. Yet she seemed not to have a care in the world. She smiled at me and I smiled back.

"You're doing better than ever," he laughed as he playfully lifted the little girl from the table and swung her around with her giggling wildly.

I wondered how he did it. He had the reputation for being a fine, caring and patient doctor. He was an excellent diagnostician, had a warm bedside manner, and had the respect of his students, fellow physicians and staff. But on my first day with him, I wondered how he dealt with many of his patients in this inner city clinic. Most of the parents I saw were hard working and caring people. But far too many were non-compliant with their medications, an appalling number did not keep their appointments and there seemed to be a pervasive lack of appreciation and respect for the hard work and dedication of the doctors and their staff.

But I learned a valuable lesson that day. In the course of my medical career I would meet many people with diverse ethical and moral standards. My duty was to provide for their physical and emotional needs. Not to judge them.

As I looked upon the pediatrician with admiration, he set the little girl down on the floor and handed her a puzzle. He then turned scornfully towards the mother.

"You do realize that your daughter is seriously ill and came very close to dying," he chastised her, "now I am counting on you not to forget to give her the antibiotic. Do you understand?"

"Sure," she answered indifferently.

"Good," he continued, "and I want to see her in two weeks. You cannot miss that appointment."

"Can't do it, Doc," she answered, "going to South Beach."

"Going where?" he asked as his frustration mounted. Only his years of experience allowed him to maintain his calm demeanor.

"Miami," she announced, "I'll be in South Beach for a few weeks. I go two or three times a year."

"Well then," he pleaded, "get her in here as soon as you get back,"

"We'll see," she said, "I'll call you."

Despite her disrespectful attitude he calmly closed her chart and got up to leave. He was unflappable.

"Doc," she called as he walked to the door, "can you write me a prescription for Tylenol?"

He looked back at her with a stunned expression. "You can buy Tylenol over the counter," he said.

"Sure," she answered, "but if you write a prescription Medicaid will pay for it."

Something finally snapped. I swear I could hear it.

"Who pays for your trips to Miami?" he asked.

She looked stunned. "Welfare," she weakly offered.

"Well if you can afford to go to Miami," he defiantly declared, "you can damn well afford to buy Tylenol."

Then he turned his back and stormed angrily away. Her jaw dropped and she looked at me. I could only shrug. I knew there was still a lesson to be learned about tolerance, patience and respect. But maybe it would take more than just one day.

The Boxer

The cheering crowd startled me as I quietly entered the patient's room. But they were not cheering for him. They didn't even know that he ever existed.

"How are you doing?" I asked as I approached his bedside.

"Who are you?" he asked, glancing quickly at me then returning his fixated stare to a boxing match on the television.

"I'm a student doctor," I explained, "I'm working with the surgeons and was asked to look at your foot."

"Gonna take it off?" he snapped, taking me by surprise.

"I don't know," I answered, "I hope not. That's for the surgeons to decide."

From the chart notes it looked as if it had already been decided but I did not want to be the one to have to break it to him.

I had just proudly begun my third year of medical school but it was obvious that he was not very impressed. We were both in our mid-twenties but beyond that I doubted that we had much in common. It was during the 1988 Olympics and he was much more interested in watching the games than talking to me.

"Do you mind if we turn off the TV so we can talk?" I ventured to ask.

"Do you mind if we don't?" he flatly replied as he continued watching.

I grudgingly took advantage of the fact that he was ignoring me to try to obtain a thorough history from his chart. He had been diagnosed with Type I Diabetes Mellitus, or Juvenile Diabetes, at the age of seventeen. He had apparently refused to accept his diagnosis and had been very non-compliant with his insulin and glucose monitoring. He had been hospitalized several times for Diabetic Ketoacidosis and for various infections. He had nerve damage to his feet and had suffered numerous foot infections. He now had a bone infection and was likely to have his left foot and perhaps lower leg amputated.

I did not know then how uncommon complications such as these were. In my practice of several years I cannot recall even one patient having an amputation from diabetes. But in an inner city hospital it was sadly commonplace. We had catchy abbreviations such as AKA for 'above knee amputation' and BKA for 'below knee amputations' that were tossed around commonly and indifferently. A BKA would be ordered as casually as a BLT. But even then I had never seen it in someone so young.

"You like boxing?" I asked, trying to start a conversation.

"Yeah," he said as he smiled and looked at me, "boxing is my sport."

"Do you . . . um . . . did you box?" I asked.

"I was a boxer," he replied, "I boxed for six years. I started when I was eleven. Placed second in the Junior Olympics. I had a good shot at going to the Olympic Games in '84 in L.A. I might have even gone to Seoul."

"Were you that good?" I asked.

"I was real good," he replied with a confident nod, "13-1 as an amateur. I fought with a lot of guys that were in the '84 Olympics. I knew a few of the guys that are fighting now."

"What happened?" I asked.

"Diabetes happened," he replied, "kinda tough to be a boxer when you got diabetes."

"I guess you're right," I said, regretting having asked the question. "Do you think you would have made the Olympics?"

"You don't know," he shrugged, "I was good but a lot of guys were good."

His eyes became misty. "It was my dream," he added.

Our conversation moved comfortably after that as we talked about boxing, the 1988 Olympics and eventually his own medical history. He politely cooperated with my examination. When we were finished we shook hands and I wished him well. I felt like I had made a friend. As I left, I was filled with sadness as I turned back to see the light of the television filling the emptiness in his eyes as he sat alone in the darkened room. He looked so isolated. He looked so forgotten.

He might have been an Olympic champion. He might have stood on the platform with a gold medal around his neck as they played the National Anthem. He might have listened to the cheers of the crowd as he basked in glory in Seoul, South Korea.

Instead he waited for an unknown doctor to amputate his left foot in a lonely hospital room in Cooper Hospital, Camden.

3

Struggles

Only Life He Had

"H-H-How . . . are . . . you . . . doing . . . to . . . day . . . Doc?" he struggled to ask me as I entered the room.

He weakly raised his right hand, which I grasped firmly to greet him.

"Good, thanks," I answered with a smile, "How are you?"

He slowly nodded and smiled weakly. He then pressed the hand control of his wheelchair to back himself to where I could check his blood pressure.

Conversation was painstaking, but I tried my best to give him the time he needed. The mere sight of him stirred compassion. Twenty years ago, he was a handsome young college student and an excellent swimmer. One Saturday night, he took a drunken ride home from a party with a friend. He lost control of the car and was involved in a horrific accident. He suffered a broken neck and head trauma resulting in severe neurological damage. His friend was pronounced dead at the scene.

He was paralyzed from the chest down, and had only minimal strength in his arms. His speech had been affected and after years of therapy could only speak very slowly and with great difficulty.

He was fortunate to have parents who were in good enough health to care for him but he still required a home health aide seven days a week. Every day of his life was a physical, mental, and emotional struggle. He could do very little for himself and was totally dependent on others. Eating, drinking, bathing, using the bathroom, and getting in and out of the wheelchair required assistance.

His eyes followed me intently as I checked his blood pressure then moved to examine him. I listened closely to his heart and lungs. I moved his frail body to inspect his skin for sores I knew he would never feel.

"Everything looks fine today," I explained, "except for your blood pressure. It's a little high so I'm going to increase your medicine slightly."

"Sounds . . . good," he answered.

At times I felt so greatly frustrated. Over the years we had talked in great detail of the struggles he faced every day. I felt almost foolish suggesting that a change in his blood pressure medication would somehow enhance his life.

The physical challenges he faced were daunting. He was a prisoner in a body that he could not control. How many days did he spend dreaming of walking along the beach and feeling the wet sand between his toes or of diving in and gliding gracefully through the water as he once had? Or of just reaching out and hugging a loved one?

Even worse was the emotional burden of that fateful day. The day played over in his mind repeatedly. Why did he drink and drive? Why was it his friend's and not his mangled body beneath the sheet on that bloody highway? Even sleep could not provide respite from the nightmares that tortured him.

He struggled to accept the guilt of his friend's death and the burden he had placed on his aging parents.

But somehow he went on. He entrusted me with his life and I would take every step, no matter how small, to keep him in alive. The quality of his life would in no way diminish the value of his life.

I knew it was not the life he had hoped for. But it was the only life he had.

Iron Horse

I looked up from my desk and we exchanged awkward smiles as he shuffled past my office and stumbled on the rug as he entered the examining room.

I began seeing him several months ago when he was having some trouble swallowing. He told me it was not severe but that his wife had noticed him choking frequently and thought he should have it checked out. I did an upper GI series that was essentially normal and he told me that he thought he was getting better.

One month ago he came back in to see me. He was a powerful man who worked as a welder. He complained that he did not feel strong anymore. He was dropping things and his muscles felt stiff and weak. He tried to minimize the problem but I could read the concern on his face.

I had sent him to a neurologist and ordered some further tests. I read the report slowly one last time before entering the room, hoping against reason that the seventh time would be different than the sixth. It was the worst part of being a doctor. But he was anxiously waiting, and it was time to discuss the results.

I remembered years ago sitting in a similar room with my mother as she was told she had colon cancer. President Reagan had been diagnosed with colon cancer at the same time and the news was full of how good his prognosis was. I took solace in the fact that my mother had the same disease as the President of the United States and I knew that they would both do well.

I have found that my own patients have been reassured to know that they were not alone in their sickness, especially if they shared the same disease with someone who was well known and enjoying an active life despite their illness. I have comforted patients who have been diagnosed with a heart condition, atrial fibrillation, by telling them that former President George Bush and former Senator Bill Bradley share the same condition.

I remember sitting in a hospital room with seventeen year old basketball player who had just been diagnosed with diabetes. He was worrying about his future basketball career and I reminded him of the inspirational story of Bobby Clarke who despite being diagnosed with diabetes at age fifteen went on to a storied NHL career which included three Most Valuable Player awards, two Stanley Cups and enshrinement in hockey's Hall of Fame.

The letter from the neurologist was fairly conclusive and left little room for hope. He had undergone a thorough evaluation, an MRI of his brain, a lumbar puncture and an EMG. The results showed a loss in function of his motor nerves consistent with amyotrophic lateral sclerosis. My mind wondered momentarily as I searched for the right words to say.

I thought of telling him that he had hit 493 career homeruns and 1,990 RBIs. Or that his teams had won six World Series championships. Perhaps it would encourage him to know that he had played through concussions and broken bones to establish a record of 2,130 consecutive games that stood for almost 60 years. Or that he was known as the Iron Horse and the Pride of the Yankees.

But as I entered the room, I knew that none of those things would really matter—not when you are forty-one and your doctor tells you that you have Lou Gehrig's disease.

Why Do You Want To Be a Doctor?

"Why do you want to become a doctor?"

The question from my medical school interview haunted me as I walked through the cheerfully decorated lobby of my patient's nursing home. I can remember with striking clarity sitting nervously across the desk from my interviewer as he posed this question. It was the first question he asked and would set the tone for the entire interview.

I shook the thoughts from my mind as the elevator door opened and I made my way to the nurses' station. I quickly found my patient's chart and began looking through it when I noticed the nurse standing before me.

"He's the same as usual," she explained with a shrug, "certainly no better. His sugar has been running high, about 250, and his blood pressure has been somewhat out of control."

I thanked her for the input and slowly walked down the dreary hall towards his room. He seemed to sense my presence as I entered and began screaming.

"My leg. My leg. My leg. My leg," he shouted. "My leg. My leg."

He was a ninety-year-old man with multiple medical problems. He suffered from high blood pressure and diabetes. His diabetes had left him nearly blind and had necessitated his left leg being amputated below his knee. He had had a stroke five years ago, which paralyzed his right side and robbed him of his speech. The only thing he could now say was "my leg", which he said loudly and repeatedly.

I never knew him as anything but this. I didn't know what he had done for a living or where he had lived. His chart listed him as widowed but that was sadly the only thing I knew about his personal life. He was the source of frequent late night phone calls from the staff and I constantly had to adjust his medication. He always seemed angry. He seemed to hate everyone. I always tried to provide sound medical care but could not help but think of him as a burden. To me. To the staff. To society.

As I approached his bed, the stench of his diaper was nauseating and I wondered when he was last changed. I walked to the left side of his bed and drew back his covers. I firmly rested my hand on his left arm as I began to examine him. I had found out the hard way that his age and failing health had done little to diminish the power behind his left hook.

As I examined him, his eyes narrowed as he stared at me. I forced a smile and tried hard not to imagine what he was thinking. I glanced around the room. There were no pictures, no cards, no flowers. The only relative listed on his chart was a nephew who lived out of state. I looked out his window at the rest of the world. People working, playing, laughing, loving. Every one of them oblivious to this forgotten soul. He had outlived life. The only thing he had to look forward to was death and it was my responsibility to do everything I could to prevent even that.

When I finished examining him I returned to the nurses' station to write some orders. I increased his insulin to better control his diabetes and added a new medicine for his blood pressure. I then quickly made my way down the hall to escape the confines that I knew my patient would never leave.

Why did I want to become a doctor? During that interview, so many years ago, had I envisioned the efforts I would put forth to prolong an existence that had long ago ceased being a life. Where his only hope could be to die and escape the deplorable conditions in which he had spent so many years. Where he would spend the rest of his days wallowing in his excrement, shouting nonsensical phrases, forgotten by the world, and void of any shred of human dignity.

"Why do you want to become a doctor?" my interviewer asked.

I cringed as I remembered my answer.

"To help people."

Dead Man Walking

Dead man walking.

The words struck me as I looked up from my chair to see him laboriously make his way past me and towards the examining room.

"Hey, Doc," he said with a strained smile as our eyes met.

"Hi . . ." I feebly replied. I could not bring myself to say "Good morning" or "How are you?" I fought to maintain my composure as I watched him struggle into the room and drop his body into the chair. Dead man walking. I shook the thought from my mind but it would not leave. He was firmly in that grip of death from which medicine was powerless to free him. I knew it. He did not.

I picked up his chart and noticed that he had lost another six pounds in just five days. I had seen him the week before for the first time in over six months. He had lost thirty pounds. He complained of fatigue and loss of appetite. His abdomen was distended and his liver had an irregular feel to it. He looked old, sick and tired.

He had been one of the healthiest eighty-five year old men I had ever known. His face had barely a wrinkle. He traveled frequently, loved to fish and bowled twice a week. He was a pleasure to talk with. He was always upbeat, enthusiastic and never failed to ask me how my family was doing.

As I entered the room, his usual big grin shone across his face but it could not hide his suffering.

"How are you?" I asked as we shared a firm handshake.

He shrugged. He could not lie. "Oh, about the same," he replied.

"I'm sorry," I told him as I sat down beside him, "but unfortunately I don't have good news for you. I got your CT scan back and it shows a sizable mass in your pancreas."

He looked at me like he understood but showed no real reaction. His eyes were wide and he reminded me of a frightened deer that was caught in the headlights. He had nowhere to escape. I wanted to stop but I couldn't.

"It also showed several tumors in your liver," I slowly continued, "some are quite large. I have to tell you that the most likely explanation for this is pancreatic cancer that has spread to your liver."

"What do I do, Doc?" he struggled to ask.

There was a trust in his voice that had grown over several years. He was one of my first patients during my residency. He lived not far from me and I remember once while in the grocery store hearing his booming voice call "Dr. Marzili". "This is my doctor," he had said as he introduced me to his wife. It was the first time I had ever run into a patient in public and it gave me a sense of pride that I will always remember. It was also the first time someone identified me as "my doctor". The words meant a great deal to me when he said them. They mean a great deal today.

"You have a choice," I explained, "I can send you to the oncologist and we might want to biopsy the mass to find out what it is. The cancer specialist may offer you some treatment, maybe chemo or radiation."

Hearing myself say it did not make it any more convincing. He was living and breathing before my eyes but I could not deny the fact that he was dying.

"Or," I added, "we can do nothing. I can try my best to make you comfortable and hopefully you will do well for some time."

He looked overwhelmed and tears formed in his eyes. "I don't know what to do, Doc," he pleaded, "you tell me what to do."

I was moved by the faith with which he placed his life in my hands. I almost always get a specialist's opinion and weigh the various options. I just wanted to do what was best for him.

"My friend," I said as I patted him reassuringly on the shoulder, "I'm not going to put you through anything else. I'm going to call a nurse to go see you. We'll try to make you comfortable and keep you active for as long as we can."

He smiled and shook my hand gratefully. My heart was heavy as I watched him agonizingly make his way from my office. Somehow I would get through the rest of the day but I felt only sadness and a profound emptiness deep in my soul. I felt like someone had ripped out my heart. Like a dead man walking.

Mickey

"Hey, Doc, how you doing?" he said in his usual friendly manner as I entered the room.

"Good," I answered, trying to hide my apprehension, "how are you?"

"Oh, I can't complain," he said, "I'll tell you something, Doc, this is the best I've felt in a long time. The breathing is good. My energy is good. That belly pain I had in the fall is gone. A twinge of pain now and then but nothing I can't handle."

He appeared to be well as he comfortably sat in the chair beside me. He was seventy three years old and suffered from mild emphysema and hypertension. His health had been good since he quit smoking five years earlier. His wife sat in a chair by the window. She joined in our friendly conversation but seemed to sense my uneasiness and suspected that I had bad news.

He was one of my first patients in the morning following a long and fitful night of sleep. I had known him for about fifteen years. He was not only my patient but my friend and barber since the days that I had a full head of hair. He has a delightful little barber shop. An American flag flies proudly from his porch and the red, white and blue spin in the barber pole on his front yard. You wait in an orderly row of red vinyl chairs and read the morning paper or join in the pleasant banter among his customers. He decorates his house and shop with boyish enthusiasm for every season and holiday. A trip to his shop is like walking into a Norman Rockwell painting. Pictures of children's first haircuts line the wall and every customer is his friend.

Inevitably when I am there someone will say, "Hey Mickey, you're looking good." And then he will point to me and proudly say, "He keeps me healthy, this is my family doctor." There is something charming and welcoming about a visit there and I always leave feeling good.

He is semi-retired now although to him that means five eight hour days a week. But he takes more time off now for vacations and cruises and doctor visits.

"I got you're CAT scan results back," I began to explain, "and I'm afraid there were some areas of concern. There seems to be an abnormal area in your intestines and a few worrisome spots in your liver."

He looked at me with his usual trusting eyes and I knew I had to be more straightforward.

"There are a few possible explanations for this," I hesitantly continued, "but to be honest it looks like it is some type of cancer."

He looked at me and then back at his wife. He was a strong and resilient man. In addition to being a barber he had worked for several years as a policeman. While in the army he survived being struck by lightning. A few years ago he had fluid around his lungs that we feared was a sign of lung cancer. His only daughter had recently completed treatment for breast cancer. He had bravely faced every ordeal and had come through even stronger. I have known few men who were so tough yet so gentle.

I saw a tear form in his eye and I fought hard to maintain my composure as I explained how we would further evaluate and treat him. I arranged to have a biopsy which confirmed the presence of a carcinoid tumor of his small intestine and liver. I referred him to an oncologist for what I hope and pray will be a successful course of treatment.

I often wonder how the oncologists deal with it. But then every patient they see already has cancer. They walk in as a life to be saved. A burden of suffering to be eased. But as a family doctor I have forged a relationship over years and the grief is much more personal. My barber with cancer in his liver. The lovely young mother of twins who struggled through years of infertility treatment and now faces breast cancer. The delightful businessman who battled through a difficult divorce and recovered from financial ruin only to be diagnosed with leukemia. The compassionate hospice nurse with the inoperable brain tumor who now faces hospice herself.

I love being a doctor and hope to continue my career for many years to come. But sometimes I can see why doctors burn out. I can understand why they retire. I can foresee a time when I may get tired of seeing colds, hypertension, diabetes, heart disease and cancer and cancer and cancer.

A Death in Salem

"I got a complaint from a nurse on the third floor," the Chief of the Medical Staff began as my mind raced, "she thought you called a code too quickly. She said that you only tried to resuscitate the patient for about ten minutes."

He handed me the chart and sat there silently. I nervously paged through the chart as I tried to recall the case that had occurred a few weeks ago. It was a serious accusation. The nurse was apparently caring for the patient and thought I did not do everything possible to save his life. She thought that I was in some way responsible for the man's death.

The previous night had started routinely enough. I had been moonlighting as a house doctor as I had done for approximately six months in a hospital in rural Salem County, New Jersey towards the end of my residency. I had received an ominous note attached to the roster of hospitalized patients requesting that I report to the Medical Affairs office in the morning. But my conscience was clear and I thought little more about it.

I read through the chart with knots in my stomach. I could feel his eyes piercing me as I carefully read every line. I was in a precarious position. The facts of the case seemed to not matter. A man was dead. I had run the code and a nurse who was helping had thought I had not done a good job and essentially blamed me for the patient's death.

The Chief of the Medical Staff leaned back in his chair expectantly. He was an old Navy doctor who was now semi-retired from private practice but remained very active in the hospital. He was about seventy years old, with wire rimmed glasses and gray hair cut neatly in a crew cut. He stood up straight and tall and had a commanding presence. Everyone called him "Sir". He seemed like the firm but gentle grandfatherly type but I did not know him well enough to count on the gentle side.

There were many challenges one faced as a house doctor. I cared for many critically ill patients. I was often tired and frequently asleep when the calls came in. Some patients died. But as I retraced my steps in my mind I could not recall anything I had done wrong.

"It was a short code, Sir," I said as I struggled to concentrate through my fatigue. I had had a hectic night and was working on about two hours sleep. But I knew I had to face the accusation then and there. I would have to choose my words carefully. We were talking about a man's death. At stake were my reputation, my job and my honor.

"I had been called several times to that patient's room for pain," I explained. "He had prostate cancer all through his bones and for days nothing would control his pain. He was terminally ill."

As I recounted the scene I searched for the face of my accuser. I did not know the nurses at this hospital well. I remembered the incident as nothing but routine or at least as routine as a code could be. No one seemed unusually troubled. No one spoke up or gave any sign of disapproval. I knew that the nurse must have felt close to the patient and had taken his death personally. Yet I cannot describe how horrible it felt to know that she held me responsible for this man's death.

"As I was running the code," I continued, "they reached the patient's attending physician. When I told him we were coding his patient he told me that the patient had cancer throughout his body and there was little that could be done. The last thing he said was not to run the code too long. Still, I feel I did everything I could to save his life."

I had my say. Anything more would have seemed overly defensive. I sat and waited for his judgment. He nodded thoughtfully then took off his glasses, folded them slowly and placed them on the desk.

"Okay, son," he said reassuringly, "I figured there was an explanation. Go home and get some sleep."

He then closed the file and tossed it gently on top of a pile of charts on a chair.

Then he said something I will always remember. It was not particularly profound. I just remember that he said it.

"Some people just die," he said. And that was the last I heard about the death in Salem.

4

Sinners and Saints

Striking Out

I glanced at the chart of a new patient who was here for allergies. Looking at his personal information I noticed his employer was Major League Baseball. His occupation was National League umpire. Wow, I had a major league umpire for a patient. I followed baseball but did not recognize his name.

I introduced myself as I entered the room. He immediately extended a firm handshake and pleasantly introduced himself. "I'm new to the area and figured I should find a doctor before the season starts. Are you a baseball fan?" he asked.

We have some important people in our practice and I always try to keep the conversation medical and not overly pry into their careers. Others seemed reluctant to talk about their professional life and I respected that. It struck me as odd that he was so anxious to talk about his career. "I sure am," I answered.

He went on to tell me what it was like being an umpire. He described standing behind the plate watching batters trying to hit a Greg Maddux pitch. Hearing the crack of the bat from six feet away as Mark McGwire launches a long home run. Arguing face to face with Barry Bonds after calling him out on a stolen base attempt. I was mesmerized.

"Do you go to any games?" he asked, "I can get tickets right behind the dugout. I'll give them to you sometime." What a great guy.

We briefly discussed his medical condition and I examined him. I gave him a prescription for an antihistamine.

"Oh, by the way, I forgot my wallet. I'll drop off my insurance information later and I'll bring you some tickets," he explained.

This also seemed peculiar. Why would a new patient show up without any identification, insurance, or means to pay? I guess it could have been an oversight, and he was giving me tickets. And what reason would he have for being dishonest.

"One more thing," he added as I was getting ready to say goodbye, "I have a chronic back problem."

Oh, no. I had a feeling I knew where he was going. He was going to ask me for narcotics. Please, let me be wrong.

"I can't take anti-inflammatories because they upset my stomach," he continued, "and Tylenol doesn't work. My old doctor gave me Percocet. I only use it when the pain is really bad."

The suspicions I had subconsciously ignored now became more obvious. Now I saw his motive. I had wanted so badly for him to be who he said he was, but now I had my doubts.

I excused myself from the room. I sat down and pondered what to do. I called the telephone number he had given. It was not in service.

I returned to the room and explained that without any medical records, I could not give him any controlled drugs. He reasoned with me, then pleaded with me, but he could see I would not budge. Finally, he sullenly left the room.

His elaborate ruse to get narcotics from me was the best I had ever seen and I could not help but admire his effort. He was very sharp. But today, thankfully, he struck out.

Fast Track

"Excuse me, I've got to go, the doctor just came in," he said, quickly ending his cellular phone conversation. "So how are you doing today, Doc?"

He was a stylishly dressed twenty-four year old pharmacist. He was fast talking but personable. I had known him for about two years. He was very talkative and his favorite subject was himself.

"Guess what," he started, "I'm going to law school. Yeah, I just can't see being a pharmacist all my life. I have some friends who were pharmacists and went to law school and they're doing awesome. They got great jobs with pharmaceutical firms and are making some really big bucks. I'll still work as a pharmacist during law school. Not many law students are going to be making the kind of money I am working part-time."

"What can I do for you today?" I asked.

"I need this physical form filled out for school," he answered, "and I was also hoping you could check my back. It's been bothering me since I started working out at the gym. I've been using some Percs and Vals but it's still bothering me."

He was a likable young man but something about him made me feel uncomfortable. Hearing a pharmacist refer to Percocet and Valium by their street names only deepened that feeling.

I completed his form and examined his back. I gave him a prescription for an anti-inflammatory and sent him for an X-ray. He suggested a stronger narcotic but was not insistent. I wished him good luck in law school and off he went in his new BMW.

Several months later I got a call from an investigator. He asked me if I had recently written or called in prescriptions for a narcotic on one of my patients. The question surprised me. I had written the pain medicine for a cancer patient but the patient had died more that six months ago.

The investigator explained that they had been investigating a pharmacist for stealing narcotics. He had been falsifying prescriptions and altering the pharmacy records. But he had gotten careless and now faced the loss of his license and perhaps criminal charges. They were not sure if he was abusing drugs or selling them on the street.

When he told me the name of the pharmacist my heart dropped. It was the law student. I could not help but feel deep pity for the young man. He was so bright and had so much potential but had thrown it all away.

Having falsified my prescriptions, I doubted that I would ever see him again. I did not think he would ever be able to face me. Over the next three years I often wondered what had become of him. Would he ever work as a pharmacist again? Was he able to continue in law school? Did he go to prison?

I had no idea what he was doing or where he was working. Then, by chance, one day I ran into him where he was working. I thought of avoiding him but it was too late.

I knew that he recognized me but he pretended not to. He looked in my direction but avoided any eye contact. "Can I help you?" He asked in a disinterested manner.

I wanted to ask him what had happened. I wanted to ask him how he was doing. I wanted to tell him that I often thought about him and ask if there was anything that I could do to help.

But I could not bring myself to do it. So I just answered his question.

"I'd like a cheeseburger and fries."

Between Heaven and Hell

"Go do a history and physical on the new patient in 842," my resident ordered me as I began my first medicine rotation as a third year medical student.

"Oh, and be careful," he wryly added, "he's a murderer."

I was not sure if he was kidding or serious until I picked up the patient's chart and nervously headed to his room at the end of the eighth floor hall. Standing outside the patient's room were two armed guards sharing a laugh over a cup of coffee. I nervously approached expecting to be questioned, searched, or scanned with a metal detector. They barely seemed to notice me as I walked by and entered his room.

Heavy rains, thunder and lightning from a summer's afternoon thunderstorm gave the room a surreal appearance. I nervously approached the patient. He was a large man whose feet overhung the bed. He had a gaunt face and looked older than his sixty-three years.

As he lay unconscious in the bed I carefully perused his chart. Heavy smoker . . . two previous heart attacks . . . cardiac arrest . . . down ten minutes . . . resuscitated in ER . . . anoxic brain damage . . . suspected brain death. The medical facts seemed self-evident. All that was left was to examine him thoroughly, review his tests, and then write up the report for the chart.

As I began examining him, I could not resist being drawn by a deep interest in who the man was. Several tattoos covered his body and all the more heightened my curiosity.

On the fingers of his left hand were the letters L-O-V-E while his right hand contained the letters H-A-T-E. On his left arm were the letters U.S.M.C. and the Marine Corp's insignia. Below this were listed the names of several Philippine cities. I wondered how long he had served in the Marines. Had he been hardened by the horrors of war or perhaps tortured in a prisoner of war camp?

His right arm contained a large heart with the name "Josephine" and beneath that were two small hearts with the names "Mary" and "Anthony". I assumed this to be his wife and children. I wondered if they were still in contact with him. Did they know he was dying? Did they care? I shuddered as I wondered who it was he had killed.

As I began studying his chart, I was struck with the realization that the understanding of the human body could be within my grasp. Not so the soul.

As I sorted out the medical facts, my mind raced in wonder of the man not only as my patient but also as a soldier, a husband and a father. And as a killer. I wondered about the love and the hate, the goodness and the evil that possessed his now dying heart.

I looked out the window as the storm moved away, lighting up the city skyline. Far below my eighth floor window, I watched the water as it rushed off the streets and was sucked down the storm drains through subterranean passageways as it made its way to the river's depths.

I looked at my patient's face and imagined him as a much younger man as the judge sentenced him to life in prison. Now unbeknownst to him, his sentence was nearly complete. Had his debt to society been paid in full?

From the eighth floor window, I looked up to see the storm clouds breaking up. Beyond them, blue sky, and beyond that, heaven.

And as I sat alone with the dying murderer, I wondered if the eighth floor was as close as he would ever come.

His Recovery

They had been my patients for as long as I had been a doctor. They were a wonderful older couple, the kind of patients that made the practice of medicine a pleasure. I looked forward to their visits. They would always come in together. They would dress up nicely and be extremely loving towards each other.

They were generally in good health and rarely complained about anything. Their visits sometimes seemed more like social visits than medical encounters. They would come in late in the morning and after seeing me would always go out to lunch together. They were thoroughly enjoying their retirement years.

I feared that would all change one Sunday morning when he called me complaining of chest pains. They called an ambulance and rushed him to the hospital. He had suffered a heart attack. To my amazement, when I saw him back in the office two weeks later he looked like his old self again. His wife had taken marvelous care of him and he was determined to make a swift and full recovery.

Two years later, everything did change. I will never forget the look on their faces when I told them that she had a mass in her lung. She too was determined to recover but it was not to be. She died a few short months later.

I was worried about him after his wife died. They had done everything together and now he was alone. He was depressed as expected but I was pleased to see the sparkle return to his eye a few months later as he again seemed to take pleasure in life.

"Doctor," he said at the end of a visit about a year after his wife died, "I saw a commercial on TV about Viagra and it said that you could ask your doctor for free samples."

We talked briefly, and I gave him some samples and a prescription. He returned to my office about two months later.

"Doctor," he said with deep sincerity at the end of the visit, "I really want to thank you from the bottom of my heart for everything you've done for me. I was devastated after my wife died. We had a wonderful marriage. I'm seventy-four and after I lost her there were certain pleasures in life that I never thought I would experience again. Because of your help, I now can and I'm very grateful."

He warmly shook my hand then reached out and hugged me. The genuine happiness on his face had been reward enough. It was one of those moments that make the medical profession so rewarding, that make me so proud to be a doctor. I could have taken that moment and held it in my heart and treasured it all day, all night, all week.

But no, I was not wise enough to do that. I had to push it, I had to bask it the spotlight, I had to ask another question.

"So," I asked, "you must have found someone very special?"

The palpable silence that followed let me know that I had asked one question too many.

"Not really," he shrugged, "just hookers."

Where was Junior?

What happened to Junior? My mind raced for the answer as I gently handed her a tissue to wipe away her tears.

We had just finished reviewing her labs. She was a seventy year old woman who suffered from diabetes but was generally doing well. Her most recent labs had shown her diabetes to be very poorly controlled. All I had asked her was if anything had changed.

"I can't do it without my son," she cried, "He did everything for me. He bought my medicine for me, he helped me inject my insulin and check my sugar. He drove me to the lab and to the doctor's office. Once I lost my syringes and he tore the house apart looking for them. I'm so lost without him."

"I'm so sorry to hear," I offered.

Her overwhelming sense of loss wore deeply on her face. I wanted to say more but did not. Should I have known what had happened to him? Should I ask? She had been overdue for this office visit, presumably because her son could not take her, and I wondered if she had mentioned something about this before. Had he been ill? Was he in some sort of an accident or suffer a fatal heart attack? I often make a note of a family member's illness in my chart but her previous office note had none. I vaguely remembered her mentioning a son with a drug problem but could recall no more.

"He was such a good boy," she sadly continued, "a mother couldn't have hoped for a better son. Oh, he had his problems, but he did everything for his mother. That's why my sugar is so high now. I don't have him to help me. I just don't care any more. I don't have anything to live for."

There was an air of hopelessness in her tone that worried me. I studied her as we sat in silence except for the quiet murmur of her weeping. Her hair, which was usually meticulously groomed, was uncombed. Her clothes looked like they had been worn for days. Her constant tears accentuated the deep wrinkles that lined her face.

"You still have the rest of your family to live for," I said.

"I know," she replied as she smiled softly, "I'm not suicidal or anything. My son would never want me to do that. I pray a lot. I know that God will help me and my family get through this. God blessed me with a wonderful son for forty-eight years and I'm so grateful for that. I'll be strong for my son's sake."

"It's good that you have your religion," I said.

"Oh, yes," she replied, "I never miss Mass. My son used to take me every Sunday."

As she continued to talk about her son, I began to appreciate what a wonderful person he had been to her. He sounded too good to be true. But somewhere in her words along with attending Mass, helping the neighbors and looking for syringes I must have missed something. It must have been in her words or in her inflection. But I was caught up in her loss and I didn't hear it.

"I just miss him so much," she concluded as she gently shook her head and looked up towards heaven.

"I'm so sorry for your loss," I said as I reached out and softly squeezed her hand, "sometimes we just don't understand why God takes our loved ones away."

She looked squarely into my eyes with a perplexed and slightly embarrassed expression.

"God didn't take my son away," she said, "he went to jail for armed robbery."

The Saint

I hesitated and drew a deep breath as I prepared to enter the room. It wasn't that she was a difficult patient. I just never quite knew what I was walking into.

"Good afternoon," I said as I entered.

She was sitting passively in the chair with her hands folded on her lap. She slowly and stiffly turned her body towards me. She looked up at me with surprised recognition.

"How are you, doctor," she enthusiastically said, "it's wonderful to see you."

I imagined that it was wonderful for her to see me. After spending three months in a psychiatric hospital, she must have been thrilled to reenter her former life. She looked well as she sat before me and wore a peaceful expression. The last I heard from her she had been running naked down her street. The CIA was trying to assassinate her. At least that is what she told the doctors in the emergency room.

"You look great," I told her, "I can't remember the last time you looked so well."

"Well, I am," she enthusiastically interrupted, "my psychiatrist has me on a new medication and I'm doing great. I don't want to have to go back to the hospital."

I scanned through the summary of her hospital admission. The report said that she suffered from Paranoid Schizophrenia, with delusions of grandeur and delusions of persecution. As a doctor, I well understood these descriptive terms.

Her family did not understand. They said she was crazy.

She was a fifty-four year old woman. She had a hard life, was a heavy smoker and had deep wrinkles and unkempt gray hair that made her look much older. She repeatedly thrust her tongue in and out of her mouth and moved her hands and arms in an odd manner. These were common side effects of her anti-psychotic medication but to the untrained eye gave her a bizarre appearance. Even in a crowded waiting room, no one ever sat next to her. No one.

"Is everything going well?" I asked. I was pleased with the visit and began to hope that at last she had really turned the corner and would do well.

"Yes," she said with a satisfied smile, "I'm a saint."

"Uh . . . what do you mean by that?" I hesitantly asked.

"I'm just a saint," she explained, "nothing crazy. I can't do miracles or anything like that. I'm just a saint."

"Does your psychiatrist know that you're a saint?" I asked.

"Yes," she answered, "but I'm not sure he believes me. I'm going to see him tomorrow."

I continued to talk to her and examine her. I was concerned that she may still be delusional but satisfied that she was seeing her psychiatrist the next day. I shook her hand and turned to leave.

"Do you want me to bless you?" she asked.

I hesitated and looked into her pleading eyes. I knew I shouldn't. To do so would validate her delusion. But I had seen her chased by the CIA, be the target of a mafia hit, and be poisoned by the lady at church over a disputed parking space. This just didn't seem very harmful.

She placed her hand on my shoulder and rambled through some disjointed prayer. She wore a look I had never seen from her before. In her face I saw serenity and pride in the confidence I had placed in her. Then she smiled. And I felt blessed.

5

Time and Compassion

My Time

I glanced at my watch as I picked up her chart

"Good afternoon," I greeted her as I entered the room.

"Good afternoon Doctor," she replied as her eyes lit up. Her spirit seemed to rise from the wheelchair to greet me but her body was not willing. "How have you been?" she asked. "And how are those beautiful little children of yours?"

I studied her frail body as we engaged in our usual cheerful small talk. She was impeccably dressed as always and her hair was flawless. She was seventy-seven years old and in spite of her meticulous care looked even older. Conversation was painstaking as she paused to take a breath every three or four words.

Years of smoking had taken their toll on her body. Deep wrinkles lined her face. Plastic tubes carrying life-sustaining oxygen wrapped around her ears and into her nose.

She sat comfortably in a wheelchair. Severe debilitating arthritis and a broken hip from which she never completely recovered made walking almost impossible. Still she persevered. In the three years that I had known her she had remained relatively stable.

She had led a rich full life. She was a New York City native who followed her father into the newspaper business and had a successful career in her own right as an editor for a New York City paper.

She had enjoyed retirement until four years ago when a fall resulted in a broken hip. Unable to live alone, a well-meaning daughter welcomed her into her home. While her daughter took good care her, she often felt alone and isolated from her previous life and friends.

I listened closely to her heart and lungs. She was doing well but I knew that the slightest infection could be her demise. For her own protection, her daughter rarely let her leave the house.

She quickly answered questions regarding her health, minimizing her concern. She told me that she hoped to visit New York this summer, though we both knew that it would never happen.

My receptionist paged me to the phone. "Doctor, your getting a little behind and a few patients have complained. You've been in the room for half an hour."

Despite the length of her visit, I could not help but feel badly as I concluded her appointment. "Well, Doctor, I know you have patients waiting so I'll let you go," she said as she reached her arms towards me. I bent over and gently kissed her cheek as I felt her feeble embrace around my neck.

I would have done anything in my power to help her walk again and to restore her lungs so that she could breathe freely. But I had long ago given up any delusions of ever being able to significantly improve the quality of her health.

Yet I knew that the only time she left her house was to see me. I was essentially her entire social life, her best friend, and the only person left to listen to her stories and her concerns. Our visits had become more like social calls. Of all the sophisticated medical treatments available, there was only one thing of value that I could give her. And that was my time.

I Killed a Man

"So, how high is my PSA this time," he passively asked after we exchanged greetings.

I slowly paged through his lab work although I remembered the number from seeing it the day before.

"A number is not that important," I answered, "we already know that you have prostate cancer and that it is in your bones, but it's still a slow growing cancer and you seem to be responding to treatment." I had long ago stopped ordering his Prostate Specific Antigen. It is an excellent test for detecting an early cancer or following the progress of treatment but in his advanced stage had no real value. But every time I gave him a lab slip, he would check off the PSA himself. It served only as a rising sentinel of his worsening cancer and his impending death.

"I guess you're right," he replied expectantly, "but what is it?"

"184," I reluctantly told him.

"It was 128 last time," he solemnly replied as he slumped in his chair. "It's getting pretty high isn't it?"

I shrugged. It was actually one of the highest I had ever seen. "The important thing is how you are feeling," I offered.

"I'm in a lot of pain," he answered dejectedly, "the medication helps for a while, but it doesn't last long enough."

"Let me increase the dose," I offered.

"No," he replied, "not yet. I can take a little pain."

"How are you holding up emotionally," I asked, "you've been through a lot."

"Oh, I'm okay," he replied with unconvincing bravado, "I'm not afraid. I'm not afraid of dying." He looked me in the eyes as if to see if I was persuaded. Then he looked down and continued talking. "I've been through a lot in my day. I've seen people die before. I killed a man myself."

We both sat for a moment in silence. His words took me by surprise. More noticeably, they took him by surprise.

"What happened?" I timidly questioned.

"I was in Korea," he slowly answered, visibly shaken by the memories, "I was just a kid. We were caught in an ambush. It was the first time I actually saw combat. But they didn't realize how many of us there were and we quickly overwhelmed them."

"I came face to face with a . . . with a Chinese soldier," he continued as he rocked slightly in his chair, "he shot first but he missed me. Man, did he have scared look on his face. I just started shooting like crazy. It didn't seem real. It still doesn't."

He stared at the floor as emotions flooded his face.

"He was about my age," he continued, "I was so excited at the time, real gung-ho. But he was doing his job just like me. I don't feel guilty about it. I know he would have done the same to me."

His eyes seemed to stare off in the distance. "I can still see him lying there, though," he continued, "he was making a gurgling sound. I thought of shooting him again . . . ending his misery. I just couldn't do it. I just stood there and watched him die. It was a bitter cold day. He just died there. He's been dead for fifty years. It could have just as easily been me. I never saw anyone die before. When it was all over, I found out my best buddy had gotten killed. I never felt like talking about it again. My wife knew. But nobody else. I just live with it."

We were both emotionally drained as we shook hands to say goodbye. He thanked me for listening. I sensed that it was something he had needed to get off his chest. I would not be able to stop his cancer or slow the tide of his rising PSA. I could not relieve the physical pain of the many tumors that riddled his bones. But as my dying patient held onto my hand on that somber afternoon, I knew that by at least some small measure I had eased the burden of my suffering fellowman.

Being There

When I found a nodule on his prostate, I knew exactly what to do. I referred him to the urologist who diagnosed and treated his prostate cancer.

When he came to me complaining of shortness of breath and cough, I convinced him to quit smoking and improved his breathing.

When he came to me with chest pain during exertion, I evaluated him and found out he had heart disease. He ended up with bypass surgery but his prompt treatment saved his life.

Whatever his complaint, I had been able to assess and treat him promptly. He trusted me with his life and I had not let him down. He was a robust seventy-year-old man who enjoyed his life and did not let health problems get him down. He dressed impeccably and had a wonderful sense of humor. He lived an active life, traveling and taking his wife dancing frequently.

Four months ago, he again had trouble breathing. This time his problem was more serious. His years of asbestos exposure had resulted in a rare and aggressive cancer of the lining of his lungs called a mesothelioma. He had a large amount of fluid surrounding and compressing his left lung. He was promptly diagnosed but his treatment would be much more difficult. His cancer was already quite advanced.

Within months, all treatment had failed. All the specialists that had cared for him had done everything they could. I had not seen him for six weeks when a hospice nurse called me. The specialists were through with him and he was being returned to my care during the terminal weeks of his life.

I entered his bedroom to find a pale, thin man sleeping in a hospital bed. His chest labored with the rise and fall of each breath. He smiled and weakly extended his hand towards me. I grasped his hand and held it as he drifted in and out of consciousness. I was shocked and saddened by how quickly he had deteriorated.

His wife came in and updated me on his condition. She thanked me repeatedly for coming to their house for a visit. She told me how much it meant to him for me to come out to see him. She expressed her sincere appreciation for everything I had done. Finally, it was time for me to leave. As I gently released his hand, he responded by abruptly tightening his grip and pulling me slightly towards him. He then clearly said the only two words he had said during my entire visit. "Thank you." He then released my hand and faded back into unconsciousness.

I looked up at his wife and family as they stared back at me. I felt woefully inadequate. He had put his life in my hands. I had always been able to direct him towards a treatment, a cure. But on this day there was very little I had to offer. I could only try my best to control his pain and make him comfortable. I could talk to his family and console and comfort them.

But as I looked into their eyes, I saw only serenity and gratitude. At that moment, I stopped dwelling on all the things I could not do for him and realized that I had done what was most important.

I was there.

No Time

Four dreary walls were all that surrounded me as the minutes ticked by in my patient's room. I had stopped by to see him in the rehab facility where he had spent the last three weeks since being discharged from the hospital following his stroke.

I gazed around the room and saw no pictures or flowers, only a single card signed by several co-workers with words that seemed inappropriately jovial given the serious nature of his infirmary.

As I waited for him to return from therapy I wondered how he would be and how he would react towards me. He had been my patient for years but our relationship had been tenuous at best.

He was fifty-four years old, a senior officer for a large bank. His job and his time were much more valuable than my own. I knew that because he screamed it in my receptionist's ear every time he insisted that we refill his blood pressure prescription without coming into the office to be examined and have his blood pressure checked.

"I don't have the time to sit in your office," he would shout, "I'm a busy man and can't just leave to go to the doctor. I'll make an appointment when I have time."

But he never had the time.

When I did see him in the examining room, he was always pleasant towards me. With difficulty, I was able to drag him into the office twice a year. I was less confident about how regularly he actually took his medicine.

I did the best that I could and accepted the way he would behave towards me as his doctor. I felt more sorry for his family. He had little time for them also.

His wife had finally had enough two years ago. She left with their fourteen-year-old daughter and moved out of state. Except for his complaints about child support, he expressed little regret about the demise of his marriage and the estrangement of his daughter. He had little time for them to begin with.

Our eyes met as he was wheeled into the room. His face lit up and he excitedly extended his right hand to shake mine as his left arm hung uselessly by his side. I was struck by his happiness to see me and assisted his therapist in transferring him to his bed. He solemnly described the events surrounding his stroke and enthusiastically explained the progress he was making in rehab.

As I listened to him talk, I realized that he had alienated most of his family and had few, if any, close friends. He had dedicated his time to his career and had sacrificed his family and friends. In his efforts to make a living, he forgot to make a life. I could see the disappointment on his face when I told him I had to leave and realized how much it meant for him to see a familiar face.

On my way out, I came across his therapist and asked how he was doing.

"Honestly," she replied, "not very well. He can't move his left arm at all and can barely move his leg. I'm hoping we can get him to walk with a walker but it's been slow. It's going to take some time."

And as I walked away down the lonely corridor, I realized that all he had was time.

The Fisherman

"Do you fish?" he asked as we shook hands at the end of the visit.

"Not really," I replied as he reluctantly released my hand and I made my way towards the door, "I've only fished a couple of times in my life. I'm not much of a fisherman."

He seemed lost in thought and in no hurry to end our visit. But it was a busy Monday morning and I needed to see my next patient. I wondered why he asked the question but did not have the time nor pressing curiosity to pursue it.

"Have a great summer," I added as I reached for the doorknob, "I'll see you in three months."

"Yeah, too bad you're not a fisherman," he slowly continued, "I could give you a real good deal on some fishing rods. Heck, I like you Doc, I'd be happy to give them to you if you could use them."

"You're in good shape," I told him, "why don't you use them yourself?"

"I love to fish, Doc," he said, "but it don't look like I'm going to get much of a chance to fish anymore. I used to go fishing every week for years. But not any more."

He was an eighty year old man who was in great condition. He struggled after the loss of his wife to a stroke six years ago but was again active and full of life. He was thin, with thick gray hair and just enough wrinkles to make him look distinguished. But there was a sadness in his eyes that prevented me from leaving. The clock told me to go but some compassionate force within me compelled me to ask: "Why not?"

"My best friend had a house on a lake," he explained, "I'd go up every week and we'd spend the afternoon on the dock or out on his boat. That was living. It was the house he grew up in. Did you know that we used to fish together on that lake when we were kids. I practically spent my summers on that lake when I was a boy. We've been friends that long. We both lost our wives within a year of each other so we've spent a lot of time together since."

"What happened to him?" I hesitantly asked.

"Cancer," he calmly replied as he shook his head, "It took him real quick. There was a real nice write up in the paper about him. He had a hardware store in town for years. Did you see the article?"

"I must have missed it," I confessed, "although I usually do read the obituaries."

"Me too," he laughed, "I used to always read them to see if anyone I knew died. Then I realized that everyone I knew had died. So I stopped reading them. But he was a real character. On a nice Friday afternoon he would hang a 'Gone Fishing' sign on his door and close his store. You would have liked him, Doc. Everyone did."

He continued to reminisce about his recently departed friend as I sat there ensnared in a conversation that I could not escape. He was a lonely widower whose friend had helped him through the loss of his wife. He now needed someone to help him through the sadness of the loss of his lifelong friend.

I looked at my watch as I settled back into the chair. I had dozens of things to do that were more urgent. But none that were more important.

6

Frustrations

Seeking Viagra

He was here for one thing only. "I want a prescription for Viagra."

I told him I wanted to ask him a few questions first. "Okay, but I'm as healthy as a horse and haven't needed a doctor in over twenty years," he defiantly responded.

He was fifty-two years old but could have easily passed for sixty. He was more than a little overweight. He had not shaved in a few days and had a disheveled appearance. He was obviously not trying to impress me with his grooming or hygiene. A pack of Marlboro adorned his shirt pocket. I did not smell the cigarettes but it was hard to notice anything through the strong aroma of alcohol.

He denied having any medical problems and took no medications. He remembered that his mother took insulin for diabetes. During a review of his current medical condition he admitted to recently experiencing more frequent urination and some weight loss. "My trousers have been getting loose and I've been peeing a lot, sometimes I have to get up four or five times a night to go to the bathroom."

With his increased urination and weight loss, I suspected he might have diabetes. I asked if his thirst was increased. Actually, I asked how much he was drinking. "Usually about six or eight beers a day, maybe a little more on the weekend or if there's a game on," he replied. "But some days less," he was quick to add. I suspected those days were few.

When I clarified my question he acknowledged that his overall thirst had been increased. But I did make a note of his original response.

His exam revealed an elevated blood pressure of 184/104. His liver was somewhat enlarged. A urinalysis revealed a large amount of sugar. Otherwise, his exam was unremarkable.

"So how 'bout the prescription, Doc," he asked.

I sat him down and talked to him. I told him there were many reasons for his problem that needed to be addressed. He had high blood pressure, diabetes, smoked and drank excessively. While I would hopefully be able to treat his impotence, we first had to investigate and treat his more serious problems. I gave him a slip for lab work and told him to return next week. With a disappointed look, he took the lab slip, shoved it in his pocket and walked out the door.

After he left I was quite proud of myself. He had come seeking one thing and I had diagnosed a number of more important and life threatening conditions. I was now his family doctor and we would work together to restore him to good health. Yes, it was a good thing he had come to see me.

He never came back.

The Last Cigarette

"I've had my last cigarette," he said as he mournfully left his father's hospital room. Three days later he was smoking.

That day had occurred twenty-five years ago as he left his father's deathbed. He was only twenty-eight years old. His father had smoked all his life and was now tragically dead of lung cancer at the age of fifty-six.

Two years later his wife was pregnant with their first child. He had been close to his father and was saddened that his father would never see his first grandchild. He vowed that the same thing would not happen to him.

He swore he had smoked his last cigarette as he held his beautiful baby daughter for the first time. Four months later he was smoking.

Three years later his wife was pregnant again. She too struggled with smoking and could not quit during this pregnancy. When his wife was seven months pregnant he had lost an uncle, another smoker, to heart disease at the age of fifty-four. He was now very determined.

"I've had my last cigarette," he said as he placed a small ball and glove in his son's bassinet. Six weeks later he was smoking.

He was forty-four years old and coaching his son's little league game when he began clutching his chest. He was having a heart attack. With his family anxiously looking on, he was whisked away by ambulance to the hospital. After a few long and frightening days, he was stabilized and eventually was able to go home. The cardiologist told him bluntly that if he resumed smoking he would die. His wife assured the doctor that they would both quit.

He gratefully shook the doctor's hand and promised he would not let him down. Eight months later he was smoking.

As the years passed, his wife resumed smoking. When his children were in their teens, they too began smoking.

When he was fifty-three, he was rushed to the hospital after suffering a seizure at work. He was surrounded by his wife, his now pregnant daughter, son-in-law, and son as I entered the room. Their eyes filled with tears as I explained the situation to them. The years of smoking had resulted in lung cancer. The CT scan of his brain showed that the cancer had already spread to his brain and had caused the seizure.

I told him that an oncologist would see him tomorrow and I briefly explained what his treatment options would likely be. He took my hand and thanked me. "Doc, I'll do whatever you say. I want to see my grandchild. I've definitely had my last cigarette." I saw a strong determination in his eyes and knew that this time he would not fail.

Four weeks later he was buried.

The Wrong Doctor

My curiosity rose as I picked up her chart. I clearly remembered the concern on her face when I saw her a few weeks ago and wondered what had evolved since our last visit.

She had been a very healthy, spry seventy-four year old who I saw frequently accompanying her husband but very rarely for herself. On that day however, she looked at me with grave concern. She had found a firm lump in her left breast and promptly came in to see me.

A recent mammogram had been normal, but I told her she would still need to see a surgeon and likely need a biopsy. Her daughter worked at a nearby hospital and she asked me if I knew any surgeons there.

I looked through a directory of the hospital staff. I was unfamiliar with most of the surgeons then recognized one immediately. He had operated on other patients of mine. My other patients had been very happy with him and had had good results. He had an excellent bedside manner and had always called me promptly to let me know how my patients were doing.

"I'm very nervous doctor," she said, "and I want someone who's good. Would you trust him to operate on your wife or your mother?"

I appreciated the trust that she had in me and wanted her to have confidence in her surgeon. I looked her straight in the eyes and confidently told her that I would.

As I entered the room for today's visit, she sat glumly in her chair as her husband greeted me. She had not yet had the biopsy so I was unsure what was troubling her.

"Are you okay?" I asked, "What did the surgeon tell you?"

"I don't know," she answered, looking downward. "I guess I need the biopsy." Confused, I looked at her husband who quickly answered, "She's just mad because he's a black guy."

"That's not it," she vehemently protested as she glared angrily at her husband, then quietly added, "but I think you should have told me."

"I thought he was a nice guy but she's all upset about it," her husband forcefully interjected. "I used to work with a bunch of colored guys. I got no problem with it. But it's her body and she's gotta feel comfortable with who's touching her."

I was not aware of their "criteria" for choosing doctors. I tried to convince her that he was a competent doctor but quickly realized that a lifetime of prejudice could not be erased in ten minutes.

"I'm not upset just because he's black," she tried to explain, "but I trusted you and I really think you should have told me."

I was taken aback by their reaction and struggled to respond. I explained to her the urgent need for her to have the biopsy and pleaded with her not to delay any longer.

Two weeks later I received a letter from that same surgeon. She had followed my advice and had the surgery. The lump proved to be cancer but it was in an early stage and her prognosis was excellent.

I was pleased as I read the letter and hoped in some small way that the woman's trust in her surgeon might lessen the prejudiced feelings that she had harbored all of her life.

As for me, I had violated a twisted trust that I had not known existed and I never saw them again.

The Referral

"I want a referral to an endocrinologist," he firmly stated in an irritated tone, "I called my HMO and they said I had to get a referral from you."

"Why do you need to see an endocrinologist?" I calmly asked.

"They specialize in diabetes, don't they?" he replied, "I want the best doctor available to take care of me. No offense, Doc, but your just a family doctor."

He was a fifty-four year old man who suffered from diabetes, high cholesterol and obesity. He had been my patient for years and had always been difficult. He frequently missed his office visits, rarely went for his necessary labs and seldom remembered to take his medicine. He continued to smoke despite my strong urging that he quit.

"I heard about your brother and I'm very sorry," I said, "is that why you're so concerned today?"

"He was as healthy as I am and two years younger," he answered, "One day we're playing golf together and the next day I'm making his funeral arrangements. My wife told me I'd better take care of myself or the same thing would happen to me."

I asked him to show me which medications he was taking. He pulled out a crumbled Dunkin Donuts bag and dumped them on the table. I slowly examined the bottles.

"Did you get your blood work?" I asked.

"No," he answered; "I couldn't find my lab slip."

"I started you on a new medication the last time I saw you," I continued, "I don't see it here."

"I don't remember anything about a new medication," he tersely answered.

"I haven't seen you in eight months and I know I didn't give you that much medication," I continued to question, "why do you still have so much of your prescriptions."

"I don't know," he answered with growing agitation, "my wife gets them for me. I might miss a dose once in a while. Are you going to give me the referral?"

"I don't really see why you need one," I answered, "you're suggesting that I am not giving you adequate care yet you haven't been taking your medicine, going for your lab work or keeping your appointments."

"You just don't want to gimme one because it will cost you money," he angrily answered, "I know how HMOs work. You're the gatekeeper and the more you do yourself, the more money you make."

"That has nothing to do with it," I answered, trying to stay calm, "I don't think there has been anything wrong with my treatment but you have to help. I have hundreds of diabetics and only a few need to see an endocrinologist. What is it that you think family doctors treat?"

"Colds," he answered in an obvious attempt to further antagonize me.

"You think I spent four years in medical school, three years in residency and years in practice so I could treat colds?" I questioned.

"If you're not gonna give me the referral," he replied, "I'll find a doctor who will."

I calmed down and tried my best to explain how we could better control his diabetes. But I held firm in my refusal to refer him to an endocrinologist. It was not a decision I made as a businessman or as a "gatekeeper". Maybe I was right. Maybe I was wrong. Or maybe I was just trying to be his doctor.

Chasing Ambulances

I scanned the office as I stood there waiting for the receptionist. I was in my final year of residency and was to fill in for a family doctor who was out on medical leave. He had suffered a severe leg fracture while skiing in Vail and would be missing several weeks of work.

I had only worked in our residency clinic and was quite impressed with his beautiful office. An attractive young receptionist told me that the nurse would be right with me and offered to get me a cup of coffee or a soda.

I declined and sat down in a plush chair. The office was stylishly decorated with ornate molding and wallpaper, several manicured plants, a beautiful fish tank, two television sets and up to date magazines. I looked back at his name on the door to confirm that this was a family doctor and not a specialist. Ski trips to Vail and up to date magazines. Man, this guy was living.

The nurse introduced herself, thanked me for filling in and showed me where I would be working. At the nurse's station, I looked at a schedule that was taped to the counter. The schedule appeared light with plenty of time to see patients and ample room for emergencies. As I prepared to see my first patient, the nurse taped another schedule next to the first one. This schedule was booked solid with no room for emergencies.

"Is someone else working with me tonight?" I innocently inquired.

"No," she replied, "that's the schedule for our HMO patients."

Suddenly, time became my worst enemy as I hurried off to see my first patient. As a third year resident, I knew that I would be unable to move fast enough. I saw a few patients in rapid succession. They had simple problems like colds and back pain and I began to think that perhaps I could keep up. Then as I was writing my note between patients, the nurse tugged on my shirt sleeve.

"You need to see a therapy patient," she said, "a motor vehicle accident."

I followed her down the hall to a small physical therapy room where a therapist was working with a patient.

"This is Dr. Marzili," the nurse loudly announced, emphasizing the word "doctor" and carelessly mispronouncing my last name.

"What brings you in tonight?" I asked.

"I was in a bad accident," he replied, "bad neck injury. I come three nights a week. I'm starting to make some progress but still have a long way to go."

"When did the accident happen?" I began to ask but the nurse was pulling at my sleeve before the words were completely out of my mouth.

"We already have that information," she flatly stated as she practically pulled me down the hall.

The rest of the night was more of the same. The nurse dragged me from private patient to HMO patient to therapy patient. The HMO patients could always wait. Never spend more than thirty seconds with a therapy patient.

I was too busy or too naive to comprehend what was going on at first. By the end of the night I finally realized that the physical therapy patients had to be seen so they could bill the car insurance company at the much higher fee of a doctor visit instead of a therapy visit. It was a simple system. The personal injury lawyer would refer the patient to the "accident" doctor who would run up excessive bills in a lucrative arrangement for the patient, doctor and lawyer.

I was tired as I finished the long night. The receptionist asked me when I could work again and I told her I would get back to her.

In a few short months I would finish my residency and become an attending physician. I had always felt honored and privileged to have the opportunity to enter the profession I had dreamed of since I was a child. But as I drove home that night, for the first time in my life I felt ashamed of the medical profession.

Cigarette Money

I heard the familiar hacking cough from outside the room. I had heard it so many times before that I actually knew who it was before I opened the door. It was almost ten o'clock and he was my last patient of the evening.

"Got this darn bronchitis again," he apologetically said with a cough as I entered the room.

"How long has it been going on?" I asked.

"About a week," he replied, "thanks for getting me in tonight."

He was a forty-five year old auto mechanic with a weathered face and rugged hands. He was a two pack a day smoker who I saw often. His eight-year-old son sat wearily in a chair as I examined his father. The child had long uncombed hair, a runny nose and a constant cough. It was a bitterly cold night yet he was wearing only a light jacket. I took a deep breath as I examined the patient. He and his wife were both heavy smokers. I have many patients who are smokers, but none that smelled as strong. Their clothes smelled. Their children reeked. My examining room stunk. I could only imagine what their house smelled like.

I finished examining him and stepped across the room.

"You have another case of bronchitis," I said as I shook my head, "when are going to quit smoking?"

"I don't know," he said with a laugh, "one of these days I'll have to."

I began writing a prescription for an antibiotic when he interrupted.

"Uh, doc," he said, "I'm a little short this week, you got samples of anything?"

I found him some samples of an antibiotic and returned to the room. I handed him the samples and the encounter form for the visit. He grabbed the samples then hesitantly reached for the form.

"Thanks a lot for the samples," he said, "I forgot to bring any extra money with me tonight. I don't have enough gas to get home so I have to get some gas and I have to pick up some milk for the kids' breakfast."

There was an awkward period of silence.

"Can I pay you later?" he asked. It was nice of him to ask although since he already told me he did not have any money I really could not say no. I also knew him well enough to know that later meant never.

There is something wholesome and altruistic about the practice of medicine. Like most doctors, I entered the medical profession because I wanted to help people. I would never turn away a sick patient. I think people in other service professions would be shocked to realize how much work some doctors perform without pay.

"Okay," I answered, "my receptionist will give you an envelope and you can mail the check later."

"Thanks a lot, Doc," he said enthusiastically as he vigorously shook my hand, "my wife and I really appreciate it. We'll always remember what you did for us."

He spoke sincerely yet his words had a hollow ring. I said goodnight and he took his son by the hand and walked out the door.

He may have really needed the gas and the milk or he may just have thought that he pulled one over on me. Either way, I felt good about what I had done. I tried to envision the money going for a new coat or a haircut for his son. Perhaps he would use it towards rent or food or to save for health insurance. There seemed to be no end to the possibilities for this family who could not afford the basic necessity of health care. But who was I kidding? I knew that the money would just go towards the more than $300 a month that he spent on cigarettes.

7

Mothers and Fathers

Looking for Mother

I hesitated when our eyes met and tried to suppress my shock over the elderly man's appearance. I extended my hand towards him and he weakly grasped it as I greeted him.

"This is my dad that I was telling you about," his middle-aged son said from the corner of the room.

I had not noticed him sitting there and turned slowly to greet him. I recalled our conversation a few weeks earlier. He had told me that his father had not been feeling well and asked if he could bring him in to be checked out. His words had not prepared me for the gravity of his father's illness.

His father was seventy-six years old but looked even older. His face was sunken, his muscles were wasted and his abdomen was markedly distended. His skin had a pale, yellow, waxy appearance and his eyes were deeply jaundiced.

"Could you tell me what is bothering you?" I asked though it seemed like a foolish question.

"I don't feel too good," he answered, looking at his son for help.

"Dad's been sick for a while," his son explained, "real bad for the past few weeks."

"Does he have a doctor?" I asked.

"He never goes to the doctor," his son answered, "probably hasn't been to a doctor in over thirty years. It was all I could do to get him to come in today."

"My eyes got yellow," he said, "I remember guys getting the yellow eyes in the service. I think I have hepatitis. Is that what I got?"

"Well, I don't know," I answered, "but there seems to be a problem with your liver. I think we need to put you in the hospital and run some tests."

He did not want to go into the hospital but did not have the will to resist. He was admitted that day. His liver enzymes were sky high. An ultrasound of his liver revealed several large tumors obstructing his liver. We did not know where the tumors arose from or how long they were there. But it did not matter. He had little time left and all we could offer was to keep him comfortable.

When I saw him the next day, he had deteriorated further. He was confused and appeared apprehensive. I tried to talk to him but could not engage him in any lucid conversation. Then he sat bolt upright and stared wide-eyed towards the foot of the bed and began shouting.

"Mom," he screamed, "mom!"

I followed his eyes but there was no one there. He called out again and again and began crying. He wept softly at first then began crying like a baby. He was inconsolable.

I tried to make sense of what had happened. I have heard other dying patients cry out for their mothers. Did the end of life experience rekindle a memory from the beginning of life? Was the spirit of his mother present to help him as he passed from this life to the next? Or was it simply the toxins from a failing liver poisoning his mind and accelerating his confusion?

As I entered his room the next day, he was resting comfortably and was no longer agitated. And I smiled as I realized what he had been crying for the day before. He died peacefully later that afternoon, in the loving arms of his ninety-four year old mother.

Eternal Pain

The pager startled me from a deep sleep. I fumbled about my nightstand searching for it. I looked at the clock and saw it was two o'clock on a Monday morning.

My daze cleared and turned to anger as I read the message. I immediately recognized the patient's name and was familiar with his medical "emergency". He was stone drunk and wanted to check into a rehab facility.

It was at least the fourth time over the past year that I had received this call. It was always the exact same situation. And there was always the same result.

At two o'clock in the morning there was not much I could do for him. So why did he continue to call me? I would inevitably refer him to the emergency room.

And what did it matter anyway? Within weeks he would be drinking again. Why should I again be losing sleep for this hopeless drunk?

I calmed down somewhat as I called his number. His wife was polite and apologetic. He had been drinking all day but now wanted to quit. He wanted to try rehab again.

I asked her when he was last in rehab. She told me he was there six weeks ago. I questioned his commitment to rehab and whether it was even worth going.

I was sure she could sense my frustration. I could not understand why she had not given up on him.

I advised her to take him to the emergency room as before. She thanked me, again apologized, and then hung up.

I had trouble getting back to sleep. Was I rude to her? I tried to put myself in her shoes and understand the pain she must be going through. Her husband was not a bad person. Actually, when I saw him in the office he was always a very nice man. But when he would drink, he changed.

I appeased myself by deciding to call her the next day to see how they were. Finally, I returned to sleep.

The following afternoon, I called her. She was very appreciative of my call and told me that he was in rehab and feeling well.

"Do you have any children?" she asked me. Puzzled, I told her that I have a son and daughter. "That's wonderful," she replied, "It's wonderful to have children and grandchildren as you get older. We had a son."

The last sentence surprised me. I had never known. For the next fifteen minutes she talked about her husband and his close relationship with his son. The sports, the camping trips, the fishing trips and the joy of sharing life with a loving and wonderful son. She told me about the cascade of tragic events that turned an occasional drinker into sullen alcoholic.

I was ashamed of myself for not being more sympathetic. I still did not know if I could help the man, but at least I could better understand him.

The story she told me truly broke my heart as it had her husband's spirit. The passing of years since the loss of their son had only served to further embitter him. I could not begin to fathom the hardship of their experience.

For their son's memory would not live on in his loving touch or the laughter of a grandchild. His memory would live on in the shadows of the Lincoln Memorial, as a name engraved in a cold, black, granite wall along with fifty-eight thousand other names of Americans who selflessly gave their lives in a faraway place called Vietnam.

The Boy Within

He looked up from the legal briefs he was reading and coldly nodded to me. It was his typical greeting, actually warmer than most.

His eighty year old mother was perched stiffly on the edge of the examining table while his wife stood supportively beside her. A stroke had partially paralyzed the right side of her body and impeded her speech and memory. She was no longer able to live on her own and was forced to give up her home and move halfway across the country to live with her only son and his family.

"How are you today?" I asked.

She smiled. "I . . . I . . . I . . ." she struggled to answer, then shrugged her shoulders and nodded affirmatively to let me know she was doing well. She seemed to be well though I was never completely sure. Unfortunately, I had to rely on her family. Her daughter-in-law was quite informative but her son would rarely speak.

I did not quite understand the family dynamics. To their credit, they took the woman in and cared for her when alternatively they could have put her in a nursing home. But the overwhelming impression I had from the son was that she was nothing but a burden. The few questions he would ask seemed to lack even the slightest level of endearment.

"Does she really need that lab work?"

"What, another new medicine?"

He would challenge my every move. Yet despite my concerns, she always seemed well cared for.

Weeks later, a phone call from the emergency room shattered my otherwise quiet evening. The elderly woman had suffered a heart attack. She was alive but not conscious. She had a living will that asked that no heroic measures be performed to save her life. There was little hope for survival and she was to be sent to a quiet room to spend the remaining hours of her life with her family.

When I arrived at the hospital, I was too late. Her long life had reached its conclusion a few minutes earlier. Her daughter-in-law, with teary eyes and a tissue in hand greeted me solemnly in the hall. My mind immediately wondered where her husband was. Had he worked late and not yet made it? Was he too busy? I was relieved to learn that he was there, alone in the room with his mother.

I entered quietly, unnoticed, and was struck deeply by the scene. I had only known her as a severely disabled, helpless elderly woman. He had been a dutiful son and done the right thing by taking care of her. But how hard it must have been to see his mother in such a state. He had known her as a vibrant young mother who taught him to walk, to sing, to laugh, and to love. She was the rock of his childhood, the constancy of his ever changing life who would no longer be there for him.

Perhaps he was not a cold hearted middle aged lawyer who cared for his mother out of obligation but a caring son who struggled with great difficulty to accept the aging and disability of a woman he had idolized.

As I watched him crying unabashedly with her head cradled in his arms, I realized that beneath his cold exterior beat the heart of a little boy, a little boy who had lost his mommy.

Premonition

"I am very tired, doctor," she plainly stated in her soft Filipino accent. "My husband suggests that I see you for a check up."

"How long have you been feeling this way," I asked.

"Several weeks," she answered, "it began during a trip to my homeland just before Christmas. I felt very tired when I was home. I thought it was from the trip but it has only gotten worse. Even since I have returned, I have not felt any better."

She was a captivating forty-six year old woman who had lived in the United States for over twenty years. Her husband was an American that she had met when he had traveled to the Philippines on business. She had completed college in the United States and worked at a nearby hospital as a social worker. She had two teenage sons but the rest of her family remained in the Philippines.

"I guess that must have been a pretty rugged trip," I probed.

"Oh yes, doctor," she replied, "many, many hours. I flew to Chicago then on to Tokyo, Japan. I could not get a direct flight to the Philippines. From Tokyo, it was another four hours to Manila. Once I arrived in Manila, my brother met me at the airport and we still had to drive three hours to reach my father's house."

"Did you go alone?" I asked.

"Yes, yes," she answered, "I could not pull my children out of school at that time and my husband could not get off work. It was very hectic with Christmas so close."

"Why did you have to go then?" I inquired. "Was there some sort of emergency?"

She looked at me inquisitively and seemed to be deciding whether to tell me more.

"You may not understand," she explained, "I am the youngest of six children. My father is eighty-six years old. He is very healthy for his age. His mind is very good. But he became inconsolable. He said he needed to see me. He feared he would never see me again. We respect his words. He must know that death is near. It could have no other meaning. I could not disobey his wishes. It may be difficult for you to understand but he is my father. I had no choice but to drop everything and go."

"You left your family the week before Christmas?" I asked.

"I know it may sound silly," she replied, "but our culture is much different. We have great respect for our elders."

I admired her for her commitment to her father but felt the story was somewhat curious. I have always been skeptical of premonitions. Many people have them but they are usually fueled by fear of a disease or a test result more than by any supernatural insight.

I examined her carefully. She did look somewhat pale and her heart rate was slightly elevated but there were no other abnormal findings. I sent her for some blood work but privately wondered if she was just tired from her trip or depressed about the situation with her father.

"I hope you see your father again," I said as I stood up to say goodbye.

"Thank you," she replied doubtfully, "I don't know."

I did not think much more about our conversation beyond a passing curiosity. But the wisdom of her father's words came thundering back to me a few days later when I called to tell about her test results.

Her father was never to see her again. Her tests results revealed Acute Myelogenous Leukemia. Within a few short months, she would succumb to the dreaded disease.

Perhaps her father was only speaking out of fear of his own approaching death. Maybe it was a hunch. Perhaps just a coincidence.

But her words would haunt me for a very long time and I would never again underestimate the magical bond between a father and his daughter.

Portrait of Dad

I searched for the house number as I slowly drove down the tree lined street. I was doing it as a favor to his daughter who I had known for years. I barely knew the patient. He was a seventy-eight year old widower who had lived in another state until suffering a stroke two years ago. Although he recovered well, his daughter insisted that he come to live with her.

Two months ago he had suffered a much more severe stroke. He had a complicated hospitalization during which he had suffered a heart attack and needed to be resuscitated twice.

Perhaps against better judgment, his daughter refused to give up hope and insisted that every available measure be taken to prolong her father's life. To the surprise of many, he managed to survive. Unfortunately, the end result was a man paralyzed on the right side, confined to bed, confused, and unable to speak.

She was standing at the front door as I pulled in the driveway. She warmly greeted me and anxiously led me to the living room where her father lay in a hospital bed.

"Daddy, Daddy," she shouted, trying to rouse him, "the doctor is here to see you."

His eyes moved slightly but there was no sign of recognition.

"I guess you know he didn't make much progress in rehab," his daughter said softly to me as her father silently stared at the ceiling.

"I know," I replied, "I'm very sorry." As I looked at her I noticed the great toll his illness had taken on her. The worrying had caused her to lose weight and deepened the wrinkles on her face. Her eyes were reddened from the tears but gazed at me intently, searching my face for a ray of hope.

After I finished examining him, we sat down to talk.

"Your father almost died several times," I explained, "it was only through extraordinary measures that he was able to survive."

She nodded solemnly knowing well where our conversation was leading.

"I don't know if your father would have wanted to live like this," I continued. "He is stable now but if anything happens you may want to reconsider how aggressively you want us to treat him."

As I finished talking she reached her hands to her face and began crying.

My eyes looked away from the crying woman and were drawn to an old picture that hung prominently on the wall in front of the bed. I looked into the eyes of a robust, handsome, young man who stared back at me with piercing eyes and a broad smile. His beautiful young wife sat supportively by his side and his little girl of two or three was lovingly held in his arms. The father and daughter were most striking with their faces snuggled close together and their smiles reflecting their mutual adoration. Her arms were wrapped around his broad shoulders and she was nestled securely against his sturdy chest.

Although the photograph had faded and the frame was cracked, the love and devotion between father and daughter was as alive today as it was in the old black and white photograph from more than fifty years ago.

The medical facts were indisputable. He was beyond the realm where medical intervention could make a difference. Time and disease had worn down his body and he was not long for this world.

Still I wondered if my words had been too harsh. I had known him only as a sick, elderly man who teetered on the brink of death. But she had only known him as Dad.

My Son's Questions

I slowly approached his bedside in the dimly lit hospital room. I knew he was sick. I knew he was dying. But I was taken aback by how bad he looked compared to the last time I had seen him only two weeks ago.

I glanced back at my son standing in the doorway. He was five years old and treasured Sunday mornings when he could join me on rounds. He loved the cookies and the juice in the doctors' lounge, the attention he received from the nurses and the way he could brighten a patient's day. Most of all he loved spending the morning with me and being my helper.

I had only two patients in the hospital that day. The first was a sixty-four year old man admitted for Atrial Fibrillation. He was now stable and being discharged. He loved kids and held my son on his lap. His name was Bernie. He made my son laugh when he told him that his name was like Bert and Ernie from Sesame Street and then he let my son listen to his heart with my stethoscope.

"It sounds like a clock," he gleefully laughed as he pressed my stethoscope against Bernie's chest.

But the mood in the next patient's room was dramatically different.

"This is Frank," I whispered to my son as he stared distantly at our patient, "he's very sick and I need to take care of him."

I began to regret bringing my son on this day. Frank must have been frightening to a little boy. He was dying of malignant melanoma that had spread to his liver, lungs and brain. In addition to his cancer, he had a severe case of Rheumatoid arthritis that gave his hands and fingers a twisted and disfigured appearance. His face was deeply wrinkled and pale. He stared through foggy glasses with yellow eyes. He barely spoke and struggled with every breath.

I finished my exam and wrote my note. I wondered what impression it would leave on my son.

"Is Frank going to die, Dad?" he asked.

"Yes, Thomas," I answered, "everybody dies someday. Frank is very sick."

"Is he going to die today?" he further questioned.

"I don't think today," I replied, "I don't know when he will die. Only God knows when people will die."

"He might live a couple of years then," he hopefully asked.

"No, not a couple of years," I explained, "maybe a few weeks."

"Is he going to be a skeleton?" he asked.

"No," I tried to explain. "When people die they treat their bodies so they don't decay quickly."

"But he will be a skeleton someday," he pressed.

"I guess someday," I replied.

"Did Frank smoke?" he asked.

"Yes," I answered, "but this cancer wasn't from smoking."

"Does everybody who smokes get cancer?" he inquired.

"No," I said, "not everybody. A lot do though. Smoking is very bad for you."

"Do kids get cancer?" he asked as he looked at me inquisitively.

"Sometimes but not very often," I tried to reassure him, "mostly older people."

I held his hand as we walked quietly to the car. I glanced back at him as he silently stared out the window as we drove home. Would the events of the day scar him and cause him to lose some of the innocence of childhood or would they quickly join the skinned knees, witches, monsters, nightmares, and thunderstorms and be safely tucked away in some hidden recess of his mind?

"Thomas," I said to him, "is there anything about today that you want to ask me about?"

He looked back at me with a serious gaze. Then his eyes flew open wide and he smiled. "Can we play baseball today?"

8

Love Stories

My Wife's Crazy

"My wife's crazy, she's acting nuts. She must have that old timer's disease," the elderly man complained as his wife squirmed uncomfortably in her chair.

"She's doing all kinds of crazy things," he continued, obviously angry and frustrated over his wife's behavior.

"What do you mean?" I asked.

"All kinds of things, I don't know, all kinds of things," he replied. I looked at his wife to see if I could get a better answer.

"He's upset because I took the car keys and wouldn't let him drive," she quietly answered.

"Yeah, she treats me like a child. I've been driving for sixty years and now all of a sudden she tells me I can't drive," he retorted, his anger rising.

"But dear," his wife replied, "you were in two accidents in one week. And remember when you got lost going out for your paper and the policeman had to bring you home."

"I don't remember that," he sharply responded. "And, oh yeah, she treats me terribly. She won't even let me boil water for coffee. She hollers at me like I'm a baby."

"But dear," she replied, "you started a fire in the kitchen and I just don't want you to get hurt."

"I don't remember that," he replied, "you're just making that up. You're the one that's doing crazy things."

"What can I do, Doc? Can you help me?" he pleaded, "I'm a prisoner in my own home. This woman keeps me locked up in the house all day. I'm only allowed out if she takes me out. It's terrible."

I could sense his wife's frustration and embarrassment mounting. Tears welled in her eyes.

"Dear," she implored, "the last time I left you alone I came home to find you wandering around the front yard without your pants on. The neighbors said that you went to the bathroom in their bushes."

"That's not true," he angrily replied, "I don't remember that."

He was seventy-eight years old, a retired business executive. He once had a position of great power. He was used to making decisions involving millions of dollars and hundreds of people's lives. He now struggled to find the bathroom. His Alzheimer's disease had already robbed him of a great deal of his memory.

His seventy year old wife had incredible patience. She continued to love and respect what remained of the man she had been married to for fifty years. She had a supportive family and a great understanding of her husband's disease.

Her husband, meanwhile, was light on acceptance and understanding and heavy on frustration and denial.

"I told you she was crazy, Doc," he said to me. He was pleading for me to take his side.

"I don't remember doing any of that."

'Til Death Do Us Part

I called her to offer my condolences after her husband's funeral. She was very appreciative of my call. She thanked me for the card I had sent and expressed her gratitude for the care I had given to her husband during his life and especially at the time of his death.

She was doing well. The service had been a beautiful and touching affair. She had seen friends and relatives that she had not seen in years. It was all quite overwhelming. After all, they had been married for fifty years.

Things were beginning to get back to normal. Her family had just left before I had called and this was one of the first times she was alone. She welcomed the quiet after all the hectic activity of the past few days. She had thank-you cards to write and affairs to get in order. I wished her well and asked her to see me in a few weeks when things had settled down.

I would miss their visits. He was a well-liked man who was active in his community. Unfortunately, he had severe heart disease. His lack of concern for his own health probably would have been the death of him years ago if not for his devoted wife who would dutifully make sure he never missed a dose of his medicine and called me promptly with any change in his condition.

He would likewise do the same for her. Although her health was generally good, he would bring her regularly for her visits and almost always stay with her the whole time.

Yet despite the outward devotion, deep down they simply could not stand each other. I understood it was not always this way. They used to be a happy, loving couple. But that ended many years ago.

When we were alone, he constantly complained of her nagging, how overbearing she was and how hard she was to live with. They had not slept in the same room for over twenty years. His involvement in the community was his way of getting out of the house.

I realized that the reason he always came into the exam room with her was because he was afraid of what she would say about him. And he had reason for concern. When she was alone, she would go on about his laziness and how she always had to do everything for him. She complained about how he always had to accompany her when she left the house and how she had no privacy.

It was a rather sad situation. Out of convenience, religion, limited financial resources, duty, or perhaps just habit, they stayed together.

Although I felt sorry for them, I also admired them. I knew that in their own way they did love one another. They had taken a vow and did not break it.

For better or for worse, 'til death do us part.

Every Three Months

He sat motionless on the examining table, staring down at the floor as I entered the room. "How are you today?" I asked as I extended my hand towards him.

"Good morning Doc," he answered reflexively, making a face that let me know how he was doing and that I probably should not have asked.

"Did you have a nice holiday?" I inquired, trying to coax some small talk.

"It was okay," came his curt reply.

"Did you do anything special?" I further pried.

"My son invited me over. I went for dinner but went home early," he added, "I just didn't feel like being out."

Our conversation continued with questions about his health, which were answered in a detached manner with one word replies.

I reviewed his labs with him and informed him of how well his diabetes and cholesterol were being controlled. He sat stone-faced looking down at the paper.

He sat quietly, almost catatonic, as I examined him. He was a seventy-two year old man who I had treated for years for diabetes and high cholesterol. His conditions were well controlled and he was generally in good health.

When I finished examining him, I sat him down to renew his prescriptions. I knew it was coming.

"How'd it happen, Doc, how'd it happen? I just can't stop thinking about it, Doc. I don't know how it happened."

His face was now contorted with emotions and tears welled in his eyes.

It was now my turn to sit quietly and let him do the talking.

"She was in great health. We were married for forty-five years and she was always the healthy one. She never even went to the doctor."

"We were out to dinner with my son and his wife and she was fine, she felt great," he continued.

"She had chest pain and I took her right to the hospital, right to the emergency room. The doctors said it was her heart and that it was a good thing I brought her right away. They said if I hadn't brought her she might have died. Why did they say that? I brought her right away and she died anyway."

Tears now flowed freely down his face.

"I told her I loved her and kissed her goodbye. I told her I would see her first thing in the morning. A nurse called me at three in the morning. She said my wife had taken a turn for the worse and I should come down right away. Why did she have to say that? Why did she have to lie? I knew she was dead. They said it was her heart but I don't know. I just don't know what to believe."

He blew his nose then stood up to leave. "Thanks for listening, Doc. Thank you. I'll see you in three months." He gave me a firm embrace and then he left.

He knew I had no new answers. I knew he could never resolve the questions that continued to torment him. But in the sanctuary of his doctor's office, he could express the deep emotions that he could not reveal anywhere else. I knew that in three months, every three months, we would have the same conversation as if his wife had died yesterday. Just as we had every three months for the past five years.

Memories

"Did you hear about my wife?" he urgently asked as I entered the room.

"No," I answered, somewhat confused, "what do you mean?"

"She died," he replied as he sadly shook his head, "She died. Did you know?"

"Yes," I slowly answered, "you told me. I'm sorry."

He gave an awkward smile as his eyes wandered the room. He stood up then sat back down. He and his wife had been my patients for years. It had been heartbreaking to watch them deteriorate over the past few years. His wife had suffered with many medical problems and had died of a heart attack two years ago at the age of eighty. He was eighty-three and had been in relatively good health until the death of his wife. His mind had slowly declined since then.

"I miss her," he said, "we were married for fifty-eight years."

"That's wonderful," I said, "you were very fortunate."

"I saw my mother last night," he said as if a light bulb had gone off in his mind.

"You saw your mother?" I questioned, trying to suppress my surprise.

He gave me a look as if I was crazy. "My mother's dead," he continued, "I saw my wife last night." He had a confused look as if he was trying to jar a fading memory. "She came to me while I was sleeping."

I waited silently as he stared off into space.

"She told me it was a mistake," he said as he looked me squarely in the eyes, "it was a mistake. What did she mean by that? I've been trying to figure that out all day. Was she not supposed to die? Am I supposed to be with her?"

"I don't know," I answered as I became intrigued by his story, "did she say anything else?"

"I don't remember," he replied, "but she looked happy. She looked healthy again and she looked happy. I felt better knowing that she was happy. She reached out her hand towards me. I tried to hold it but I couldn't. I just couldn't reach it."

"Fifty-eight years," he continued as a tear trickled down his cheek, "I was working in the shipyard. She was a secretary. First day I set eyes on her I knew I was going to marry her. She was twenty-one when we met. I married her six months later and it was the happiest day of my life."

He went on to emotionally detail the highlights of their lives together. I had heard the story several times before and never tired of it. I was always amazed at the clarity he retained and the passion with which he evoked these distant memories.

I asked him to have a seat on the examining table so I could examine him. He stood up and walked confusedly around the room until I gently guided him to the table. As usual, his physical exam was entirely normal.

Our conversation stretched well beyond his scheduled office visit. As I said goodbye, he held onto my hand with both of his and had a forlorn look in his eyes. I walked him to the receptionist's desk and began to complete his encounter form. I scanned the list of medical diagnoses on the form. He did not have hypertension or diabetes or heart disease or any other illness so common in men his age.

There was no room on the form to write that I had spent twenty-five minutes with him, that he had cried, or that he had revealed his most intimate secrets. I hesitated as I came to his diagnosis. It seemed an insult to him and cast a doubt on everything he had told me. But it was the only disease he had. I quickly circled the words "Alzheimer's disease" and sadly walked away.

9

Difficult Cases

The Angry Man

"How are you doing?" I cautiously asked.

"Pretty bad," he sarcastically answered, "how would you be doing if your body was full of cancer and your doctors told you there was nothing they could do?"

It was a typical answer from him and I immediately regretted asking the question.

"Is that really what your oncologist told you?" I asked.

"I don't have to tell you how doctors are," he angrily continued, "of course he used big words and acted like the stupid treatments are helping. But look at me. He must think I'm an idiot. Do I look like someone who is getting better? At the end of every visit he reminds me that I have a very serious condition and that he can't cure me. He told me I should get my affairs in order. Does that answer your question? How am I doing?"

"I'm sorry," I said.

"Well, thanks," he replied, shrugging off my pity, "a lot of good that does me."

Long before his cancer, he had been a difficult patient. He was a fifty-three year old accountant who suffered from diabetes and high blood pressure. Regrettably, we were doing a poor job controlling his diseases. He was supposed to see me every three months. Four, five, six months would pass and he would not return. Finally, I would tell him that this was the last time I would refill his medicine unless he got his labs and came in for a visit. Three or four months later I would see him. His blood pressure and blood sugar would be off the wall. He would react angrily at his test results. It was my fault. I had refused to treat him.

The cancer came as a bit of a shock. At one visit his liver enzymes were elevated. He had not been feeling well. An ultrasound revealed his liver to be full of tumors that had spread from a previously unknown colon cancer. He was quite advanced when it was discovered. Despite chemotherapy that had slowed its growth, his abdomen was now distended with fluid and his skin was becoming jaundiced.

"You seem very angry," I said.

"Wouldn't you be?" he snapped back at me.

I struggled to find a suitable response. "Would you like me to try to help you with your anger and your depressed feelings?" I asked.

"Well I think I need something," he answered as his voice softened.

As I talked to him, I noticed his mood change. I had always treated him appropriately as a doctor, but the harsh way he treated me had prevented me from feeling true compassion towards him as a person. But as he opened up to me that day, I felt a closer bond to him. We talked for a long time and I prescribed an antidepressant medication for him. As we shook hands at the end of the visit, he held onto my hand for a long time as if he was holding on for his life. Despite my firm grip, I knew that I could not save his life. I felt great sadness as I released his hand and said goodbye.

He was to follow up with me in one month. I had hoped that the medication had helped him. I believed that our talk had. I had anxiously anticipated his visit and was deeply disappointed when he did not show up. Two days later, I opened the newspaper and discovered why.

Sometimes a patient's treatment can be measured by lab tests or X-rays. Sometimes you can personally discuss their response in a follow up visit. But sometimes you just read a name in the obituaries, and you wonder if you made any difference at all.

ADD

"We had her evaluated by a psychologist who said she had ADD," her mother explained. "The psychologist recommended that she be treated with Ritalin. The psychologist can't prescribe medication though, so she said we had to see our family doctor."

The parents' faces revealed an excited anticipation for this drug that would change their daughter's and their own lives. Their thirteen year old daughter sat passively in her chair. "I brought the psychologist's report," the mother said as she proudly handed it to me, "It's very thorough."

She wasn't kidding. The report detailed the patient's medical, psychological, and scholastic history along with those of her parents and older sister. It included a multitude of psychological, knowledge and intelligence testing.

The report revealed that the child came from an intelligent family. The father taught math at a local university and the mother was a lawyer. Her older sister was an extremely bright student who was now a freshman at an Ivy League school.

But the test revealed something interesting about the girl. She was remarkably average. She achieved average scores on her standardized intelligence tests and was likewise getting average grades in school. The report revealed her to be happy, popular, and seemingly well adjusted. She just wasn't going to Harvard.

The recommendation was not exactly for the child to go on Ritalin and the psychologist did not quite diagnose ADD. She did note that the child seemed impatient and had some difficulty concentrating during the long battery of tests and suggested that perhaps a trial of Ritalin may be worth an attempt to see if it would boost her grades.

I interviewed and examined the patient. I found no evidence of hyperactivity or problems with her attention. In addition, it was obvious that the patient herself did not want to be treated with drugs. I explained that I could not honestly diagnose her with ADD and therefore could not recommend treatment.

The parents conducted themselves professionally but deep down they were livid. How dare I tell them that their daughter was average? It wasn't as if I was telling them she had cancer, diabetes, or brain damage. I just suggested that she was a normal average kid.

I felt sorry for the parents, but felt even worse for their daughter. I knew they would not let the matter rest, so I recommended that they see a pediatric neurologist who may be better trained at diagnosing and treating ADD.

I glanced out the window as they silently walked from my office. They had come seeking a drug to enhance their daughter's performance. On one hand, it was not much different than if they asked me to put their daughter on anabolic steroids so she could be a better soccer player.

And yet, I knew that their primary motivation was their heartfelt concern for their daughter and their strong desire to see her succeed. I knew they would eventually find someone to give them the drug they wanted. I wondered if they would ever come back as I watched them drive away in their car with their daughter buckled safely in the backseat and a D.A.R.E. sticker on the bumper.

Sleeping Late

"Is anybody here?" I heard him call from the waiting room of my empty office.

"Come on in," I answered as I hurried through the office to meet him.

He had come in earlier that afternoon complaining of progressive weakness in his left leg. He was a sixty-four year old retired truck driver. He smoked two packs of cigarettes a day but was in otherwise good health. He rarely came in to see me so I was immediately concerned about his complaint. When I saw him it was readily apparent that something was seriously wrong. He was dragging his left leg and walking with great difficulty.

I sent him for an immediate CT scan of his head. Although my office hours were over when the radiologist called, I knew that I could not give him this type of news over the phone. I asked the radiologist to send the patient back to my office so I could talk to him in person.

As I sat anxiously waiting his arrival, I made a few further phone calls to arrange the next steps of his treatment.

"How are you?" I asked.

"Good," he answered, "but they sure keep you waiting over there. And then they send me back here. I'm starving. I need to get home for dinner."

"I'm sorry about that," I explained, "but they did squeeze you in as an emergency."

"It's okay," he replied, "did you find out what's wrong."

"Yes," I answered, "and I'm sorry to have to tell you this but they found a mass in your brain."

"A mass," he questioned after a short silence, "you mean like a stroke?"

"No," I hesitantly explained, "I mean like a tumor."

"Oh," he replied as he casually glanced at his watch, "what do they do for it?"

"Well," I said, "I've done two things already. I called an oncologist, a specialist for this type of thing, and he will see you tomorrow. His office will call you tomorrow to tell you when to come in. I'm also going to schedule you for a chest X-ray and probably a CT of your chest. With your smoking, it's possible that the tumor started in your lungs. My receptionist will call the radiologists first thing tomorrow and schedule this for you. She'll call you after she schedules it."

I knew I had given him a great deal to digest. Breaking news like this is undoubtedly the hardest part of being a physician. But as I looked into his eyes all I could see was a puzzled expression.

"What time will they call me?" he asked.

"I know you're worried," I said, "but as soon as the office opens we will call."

"Well, what time?" he again questioned with a chuckle, "I'm retired and don't have a family so I like to sleep late, ten or eleven o'clock. Will it be before ten?"

"I don't know," I replied as he got up to leave, "maybe . . . I'm not sure. Did you understand what I told you? You have a brain tumor. Don't you think that's more important than sleeping late?"

"It's not that I'm lazy," he laughed, seemingly oblivious to the seriousness of his condition, "I enjoy retirement. I like to stay up late and read or watch TV."

I stood by dumbfounded as he slowly made his way to the door. I felt that I had failed to make him understand the gravity of his illness. Yet his medical ignorance would be the fragile shield that could protect his sanity. Over the next few weeks and months he would be facing surgery, radiation, chemotherapy, and the undeniable face of his own mortality.

And the most difficult journey of his life would begin tomorrow.

"I'll call you tomorrow," I said as a smile spread across his face, "go home and get a good night's sleep."

I Think I'm Dying

"So, do you think I'm going to die?" she asked, "Is it curable?"

"Excuse me?" I asked somewhat startled, "Going to die from what?"

"The tumors you said I had in my liver," she asked from the edge of her seat, "what can be done for them?"

"I didn't say you had any tumors in your liver," I replied, "I said you had two cysts in your liver. Cysts are common in the liver. Nothing needs to be done for them."

"So, you're saying they're incurable," she slowly responded with an air of resignation.

"No," I continued, "I'm saying they're nothing to worry about."

She nodded in distrustful acknowledgement. "I appreciate your being nice but I can take the truth. I'm going to die aren't I? I knew I had something serious wrong with me."

"You don't understand," I quickly replied, "we've found nothing seriously wrong with you. In fact, we've found nothing at all wrong with you."

I could see I would not be able to convince her. She was a thin, anxious sixty-eight year old woman who was to the best of my knowledge in very good health. She visited me frequently for a multitude of complaints. Her stomach didn't feel right, she was tired, she could not sleep, her muscles ached, her back hurt.

She had been evaluated from head to toe. Every organ had been scanned, every orifice had been probed, every imaginable lab had been checked and every specialist had been consulted.

Her insistence that she had a life threatening illness made every doctor uncomfortable and they excessively worked up every minor abnormality. She would ask several questions about any test result that was not perfect and consequently more tests were ordered.

Many specialists and I myself believed that her underlying problem was more of a psychiatric nature than a physical one. But any suggestion of the kind met with quick and stiff resistance. She adamantly refused to consider being evaluated by a psychiatrist or to be treated with any psychiatric medication.

At the end of the exhausting visit, I told her I would keep a close eye on her and watch for any changes. I gave her another lab slip and a referral for her to follow up with one of her specialists.

"Thank you," she said with a forced smile as she put on her coat, "but I still think there is something you're missing."

I watched her as she slowly made her way to the front desk. She had been my patient for years and for as long as I had known her she had been preoccupied with the belief that she was dying.

As hard as I tried to prove otherwise, I could not deny the fact that she was getting older. She had lost some of the spring from her step and her back was slightly hunched over. She was aging and as she aged I knew I had to be ever more vigilant as her risk of health problems increased. My duty was to keep her healthy and I believed that deep down all that she really wanted was to be healthy.

Still, as she looked back at me cynically, I wondered if she would have gotten even more satisfaction from just being able to tell me: "I told you so."

Bruises

"The good news is that all of your tests turned out normal," I explained as he sat calmly before me, "but unfortunately I don't have an explanation for all of your bruises."

"I think I'm fine," he shrugged, "a lot of old people have bruises. I'm a little clumsy and I just think I bruise easily".

I reviewed his lab results with him and discussed the CAT scan of his head. The labs were normal. I told him I wanted to make sure there was no bleeding in his head but even more I wanted to be sure he had not suffered a stroke that may have made him more likely to fall. He had been evaluated by a hematologist who also turned up nothing.

He was in his early eighties and was in relatively good health. Medically, his only problem was high blood pressure. The biggest burden in his life, however, was the full time care required by his wife who suffered from Alzheimer's disease. He never left her alone and provided meticulous care for her every need. She was getting progressively worse and I could see the wear on his face.

His wife sat silently in the corner of the room. I could still remember when she was a stylishly dressed, attractive woman with a warm sense of humor. She remained in good physical health except for arthritic knees for which she used a cane. She could still speak in short sentences and answer simple questions. I did not sense that she still recognized me but she seemed to at least realize that I was a doctor. I smiled at her and she smiled back.

"How are things at home?" I asked quietly. I felt uncomfortable talking about her as if she wasn't there yet I knew he could never leave her alone.

"I don't know," he replied in a hushed tone as he shook his head, "I'm not sure how much longer I can keep up. On TV they portray Alzheimer patients with grace and dignity. But I just don't see it."

"Do you have any help?" I asked. "What about your son?"

"Oh, he's a big help all right," he answered with a roll of his eyes, "he has a fit anytime I mention a nursing home but he's always too busy to help."

I looked again at his bruises. I had only met his son once and was concerned with his father's attitude towards him. I wondered if perhaps he was being abused by his son. I hated to think this, but I couldn't help wondering about it.

"Are you talking about me?" his wife angrily blurted out.

"No, dear," he calmly answered, "I'm just talking to the doctor."

She did not say another word. At the end of the visit we stood up and shook hands. I still didn't know why he had so many bruises but we were both satisfied that he seemed to be in good health.

He walked over to his wife and tenderly began to help her up.

"I don't need your help," she shouted.

He did not challenge her but turned his back to her and reached for his coat. Slowly, she raised her cane above her head and stretched her arm towards the ceiling. I stood there perplexed as to what she was doing. Then with surprising strength and swiftness she brought the cane down like a sledgehammer, delivering a harsh blow across his upper back. His eyes almost popped out of his head as the jolt was delivered. He then stood motionless for a second before his knees buckled and I grabbed him to prevent his fall. She again raised her cane but I guided him to a chair before she had a chance to finish him off.

Sometimes it takes months and thousands of dollars worth of tests to make a diagnosis. But sometimes you can find all the information you need in a few brief tumultuous moments.

The Rash

"He has this rash," his mother explained as her sixteen year old son sat passively on the examining table, "it's been there for a while and I wanted you to have a look at it."

From the look on her son's face, it was obvious that his mother had dragged him in against his will. Not unlike most teenagers, he rarely saw a doctor. He was an overweight young man with dark, greasy hair. He wore an oversized tee shirt, baggy pants and black boots. His ears were pierced, as were his tongue and left eyebrow. He had a fairly severe case of acne and I wondered if that was what his mother was talking about.

"We've got a lot of skin problems in the family," his mother continued, "my husband's father has a bad case of psoriasis and my mother had a malignant melanoma. I didn't want to mess around with this."

"What rash are we talking about?" I asked.

"Take off your shirt," his mother ordered.

He silently obeyed but I was still unsure of what they were talking about.

"Around his neck here," his mother pointed out, "this rash here."

I looked at the young man's neck. In the deep crease around his neck, there was a brown discoloration. I stepped back and examined his entire body then moved nearer and studied the rash closely.

"Does it hurt?" I asked him.

"No, man," he slowly answered.

"Does it itch or bother you in any way?" I asked.

"Maybe it itches a little," he answered, "but not really."

I pulled out a magnifying glass and slowly examined the rash around his neck. I thought I knew what it was but kept studying the rash in order to postpone the unenviable task of telling them the diagnosis.

I have had to tell people that they had cancer in the past. I have told people they had melanoma, lung cancer, brain cancer, pancreatic cancer and just about every other cancer imaginable. I have told people they had life threatening or life altering diseases like multiple sclerosis, heart attacks and strokes. And I have broken the news to unsuspecting family members about the deaths of their loved ones. I had performed those unpleasant duties many times and I was relatively comfortable doing them. But I did not quite know how to break this news to them.

I slowly walked over to my medical cabinet and methodically picked up a cotton ball and dipped it in alcohol. I firmly rubbed the cotton ball against the rash and the rash disappeared from his skin and caused a brown discoloration on the cotton ball.

I held up the cotton ball to the young man's mother. I stared at the cotton ball and could not bring myself to look into her eyes.

"Here," I said, "it's just . . ." I could not bring myself to say "dirt."

The young man appeared slightly embarrassed, his mother was horrified. I tried to maintain an air of medical professionalism as I said goodbye. I even circled the nonspecific diagnosis of "dermatitis" on his encounter form.

But I knew that this would do little to diminish the fact that his mother had just spent sixty dollars to have a doctor tell her that her son needed a bath.

Lost Pregnancy

"Labor and Delivery," came the voice from the phone, confirming my worst fears.

I was moonlighting as a house doctor at a rural hospital during my early years in practice. As a house doctor I worked through the night handling emergencies such as chest pain, shortness of breath, starting difficult IV's and running cardiopulmonary resuscitations or codes.

In this particular hospital, however, there was no in-house obstetrician. When an impending delivery arrived in the emergency room, the expectant mother would be immediately sent to labor and delivery. If the obstetrician could not arrive in time, the responsibility for the delivery would fall to the house doctor.

It wasn't that I could not deliver a baby. Throughout medical school and residency I had delivered my share. But I had not delivered one in three years and the responsibility made me nervous.

"We've got a big problem," the nurse said as my heart sank, "could you please get down here."

It was 4:00 AM as I hurriedly dragged myself through the empty corridor and into Labor and Delivery. It was a small department and appeared to be a quiet night.

"I don't know what to do," the nurse explained, "this young woman came in upset because she hadn't felt her baby move in a day and a half. She's due in two weeks. She saw her OB today and he told her that he heard the baby's heartbeat. When she called him tonight he sent her in to be checked."

"What's the situation?" I asked, unsure of what she wanted me to do.

"Her baby's dead," she said, visibly shaken, "there's no heartbeat, no movement."

"Do they know?" I asked.

She shrugged. "They know something's wrong. I don't think it should be my job to have to tell them. They're very upset."

"What about her OB?" I asked.

"He's not coming in," she said with disdain, her voice trembling. "He said there's nothing he can do so he'll see her in the morning. He's got a big Medicaid practice. He doesn't care about his patients. Do you think he heard the baby's pulse today? There's no way. He just heard the mother's pulse and told her everything was okay."

She had obviously had words with the obstetrician. As I listened and let her get it off her chest I sensed that she felt bad for having drawn me into this unpleasant situation.

"They're very upset," she warned as I made my way towards the room.

The woman was lying in her bed sobbing quietly. Her husband was angrily sauntering through the room, cursing loudly, slamming his fists down on the table and punching the walls.

"I'm gonna kill your doctor," he told her as he threw a towel across the room.

I figured he was talking about her obstetrician. But he wasn't there. I was.

He was small but muscular with deeply tanned skin and a scruffy beard. He may have been a farmer or farm laborer. I probably should have called a security guard but I was the house doctor and foolishly thought I could handle anything. I stood up straight, took a deep breath and entered the room.

I walked right up to him, extended my hand towards him and introduced myself. He glared at me.

"Are you with her OB?" he challenged.

"No," I calmly answered, "I'm just the house doctor."

I then explained to them that their baby had died and offered my sincerest condolences. I sensed that they already knew, but I had removed their last shred of hope.

The woman sobbed a little louder. I tried my best to be compassionate and professional. I tried to hide my fear. He stared at me with hardened eyes. I thought he was about to attack me. Then his eyes softened and tears began to form. He threw himself onto his wife's bed and fell crying upon her belly, upon his baby.

I thought for a moment about my own baby son, safely asleep in his crib at home. I forced the thought from my mind and threw cold water on my emotions. It was all in a day's work. It wasn't supposed to bother you.

Ten minutes later I was back asleep in my call room.

But ten years later I still remember it like it was yesterday.

10

Regrets and Triumphs

The Hug

She looked up at me and forced a smile through her tear reddened eyes. I gently shook her hand as she struggled to maintain her composure.

"It's back," she softly stated, "it's back."

"Are you sure?" I asked.

"I just spoke with my oncologist," she answered, "he had reviewed my bone marrow biopsy and said that the abnormal cells were back."

She began crying as I struggled to find the right words to say. I could not help but recognize that we were approaching the final chapters of a heartbreakingly tragic life.

Two years ago she was a beautiful and healthy thirty-eight year old woman with a ten year old son, a seven year old daughter and a loving husband. She had come to see me complaining of fatigue and bruising. I sent her for blood work that eventually led to the devastating diagnosis of acute myelogenous leukemia.

I remember talking to her husband after she was diagnosed. He was overwhelmed but remained strong and vowed to take her anywhere in the world to get her the best treatment available.

Together they faced the most difficult challenge of their lives. It would put "in sickness and in health" to the test. I suppose there are young women who would leave their seriously ill husbands. But I have never seen it happen. Unfortunately, I have seen instances where men have found their way out of marriages with seriously ill wives. During her chemotherapy, he found his comfort in the company of a female co-worker. When his wife was in remission, he left her and moved in with his girlfriend.

Thus began a bitter custody battle for their two children. Although she retained custody, her continued health problems forced the children to frequently stay with their father and as she called her, the "other woman".

"How did the oncologist say he was going to treat you?" I asked.

"He was going to call some centers where they have some clinical trials and see if I could get into one," she said as her tears began to flow freely, "he said he was still optimistic. I can't die. I have to be there for my children."

I fought back my own tears as she sat there crying. She was stylishly dressed and remained attractive and healthy looking despite what the tests said. Yet she looked so pathetically alone and vulnerable as she sat before me. She had the weight of the world on her shoulders and needed someone to reassure her, to give her hope. But more than that, she just seemed to need someone to hold her and to be there for her. A part of me wanted to hug her tightly, to let her cry on my shoulder, to reassure her and to tell her that her children would be okay. Instead, I awkwardly handed her a tissue and gently patted her hand. And I sat there with an empty feeling as she said goodbye and left.

When do you cross that line from which you may never go back? At critical times, I often struggle with finding the suitable time to express human affection or to broach sensitive topics such as religion that may give a seriously ill patient so much comfort. These things often seem beyond the bounds of a doctor-patient relationship.

As I sat with her that day, I thought that hugging her at that time would not have been an appropriate thing to do. But she died three weeks later, and I will always wish that I had.

Six Weeks

I slowly released his lifeless hand and paced aimlessly through the intensive care unit. I was emotionally exhausted and took a moment to recompose myself before talking to his family. It had been a long hard road.

The last six weeks had forged a strong bond between his family and myself. I remembered the panic stricken call I had received from his wife when he had been rushed to the hospital in cardiac arrest. It seemed like it happened yesterday.

He had collapsed in the yard while raking leaves. A neighbor was quickly on the scene and began CPR. The paramedics arrived a short while later and were able to re-establish a pulse. In the hospital his blood pressure was precariously low and he was unconscious.

"I don't know what to do," his wife cried the next morning as she sat by her husband's bedside, "I want him to live but I don't want him to be a vegetable. I know it's my decision but I don't know the right answer. I can't give up on him yet."

Despite the ventilator tube down his throat, several monitors and intravenous lines, he looked as if he was sleeping peacefully.

I had known the man since I had started in practice and I was not ready to give up on him either. I encouraged her to wait a day or two and see if he improved.

By what seemed to be a miracle, the next day he opened his eyes and seemed to recognize the people around him. But he was still far from being out of the woods. His heart went into failure the following day and it looked like he might not survive. But with aggressive medical treatment, he again pulled through.

The next six weeks were a roller coaster ride. His kidneys began failing, he developed a lung infection, his liver became inflamed and he suffered a bleeding ulcer of his stomach. Every time it looked like he might finally be turning the corner, another major setback would strike. And when these setbacks would nearly cause us to lose hope, the next day he would greet us with a weak smile and a feeble thumbs-up sign.

His will to live was tremendous and everything was done to help him. Several specialists helped care for him and the nurses and staff were remarkable. Yet in the end, the severe damage suffered by his heart could not be overcome. He again went into cardiac arrest and could not be resuscitated.

I felt terrible about his death. His family was wonderful and did as much to console me as I did them. The six horrible weeks had prepared them for his death and they were very gracious and thankful for all that his doctors had done.

As I said goodbye and walked down the darkened corridor I could not escape a feeling of deep guilt. I knew that I had helped to do everything possible to prevent his death. But as I walked through the parking lot on that cold winter's evening, I realized that the guilt I was feeling was not for his death but for the six agonizing weeks that I had fought for his life.

Mission of a Dying Man

I looked askance at the words of the letters that filled his bursting chart. Inoperable lung cancer. Cirrhosis. Hepatitis C. Alcohol abuse. Drug abuse. I tried to shake the impersonal terms as I opened the door to see a unique individual.

"It's good to see you," I said as I warmly shook his hand, "it's been a long time."

"Yeah, well, Doc," he said with a smile as he ran his fingers through his unruly salt and pepper hair, "I've been pretty much in demand by a lot of people these days. I'm just doing my best."

"Are you finished with your radiation?" I asked.

"For now," he said with a shrug, "I guess we'll see what the future holds."

"Are they going to give you chemotherapy?" I questioned.

"Nah," he said as he shook his head, "they said my liver couldn't take it. What are you gonna do? I got myself into this mess. It's in God's hands now."

He was a thin fifty-six year old man with a weathered face and several missing teeth. His skin displayed several tattoos and numerous scars. He walked with a limp from an injury suffered in a motorcycle accident and his voice was hoarse from cigarettes. His formal education had been short and unproductive. Life's lessons were learned as part of a motorcycle gang and during the many years he spent in the state prison system.

His past life's problems seemed inconsequential now. Years of heavy smoking had led him to being diagnosed with lung cancer about a year earlier. His cancer was already inoperable when it was diagnosed. His years of drug abuse were responsible for his Hepatitis C. Alcohol abuse had completed the one-two punch that had rendered his liver barely functioning.

"How do you feel," I asked, "are you still able to get out much?"

"Darn right," he said with a smile, "I'm not going to die sitting down. I've been out on the lecture circuit."

"Who do you lecture to?" I asked, thinking he was kidding.

"Kids mostly," he replied, "you know, schools, church groups. Whoever will listen. You know, Doc, I've done some pretty bad things in my life. I'm ashamed to tell you some of the things. I've done things to other people that I'm not proud of. Even worse is what I've done to myself. The smoking, the boozing, the drugs. You don't know the half of it. And what's it gotten me. I've spent half my life in prison. I ain't got no family. My liver's shot. I'm dying of lung cancer. Great life, huh."

"You don't have anyone?" I asked.

"I wrote a letter to my sister," he sadly replied, "she didn't even write back. She knows I'm worthless."

"Well maybe you'll reach some kid before he makes the same mistakes," I said.

"You got it, Doc," he smiled as his eyes lit up, "even if I reach just one kid in one lecture. Just maybe then I won't die in vain."

He then walked over to his jacket, pulled out a small bible and placed in reverently on the table before him.

"Been praying," he said solemnly, "my mom used to teach me this stuff when I was a kid. Never meant nothing to me. But it's never too late. I just hope God forgives me. Do you pray, Doc?"

"Yes," I answered, "I pray."

"Maybe you can remember to pray for me," he asked.

As I shook his hand I saw tears welling in his eyes and I softly embraced him. Most men in his shoes would be fighting for their lives. He was only fighting for his soul.

Borrowed Time

The first time I met him, he was already dead.

I was a second year resident at the time and burst from my call room to respond to an urgent page of "Code Blue". I entered his room to find the lifeless body of a frail eighty year old man. The respiratory technician was pumping air into his lungs while a nurse was performing chest compressions. "V-fib", she firmly stated.

Quickly assessing the situation I grasped the defibrillator paddles and pressed them against his chest. "Clear", I shouted, carefully watching the monitor as his chest heaved from the bed. His heartbeat was restored but within minutes he was again pulseless and efforts to resuscitate him were renewed.

Against all odds, thirty minutes later we were wheeling him down to the Intensive Care Unit. He had survived but I knew the chances of him leaving the hospital alive were still remote.

I entered the waiting room to find his daughter sitting alone with her face in her hands. She quickly stood up and rushed towards me. Her eyes were fixed on mine. "Is he . . . ?" she began.

"He's alive," I said, completing the words she could not bear to say, "but I'm afraid he's in very critical condition." I went on to explain what we had done and what we would do for him. I tried to be optimistic yet needed to prepare her for his possible demise.

Her face was drawn and her eyes were red. "Doctor," she said, "I'm sorry I'm such a mess. My mother is up on the sixth floor dying of cancer. The stress just got to my dad and he started having chest pain. But I never dreamed I would lose both of my parents at the same time. Daddy has always been so strong."

I did not know if her father was strong enough to survive, but I was determined to do everything in my power to keep him alive. The night dragged on. His daughter waited by his bedside sobbing and praying with all of her strength.

The break of dawn found him still clinging to life. Before I left for the next day, I stopped by to see them. His daughter hugged me and thanked me for all I had done and that was the last that I saw them.

Two years later, I had completed residency and taken over the practice of a retiring doctor. One evening I walked into the room of a distinguished looking eighty-two year old gentleman. He was there with his daughter and they were apprehensive about having to change doctors. The moment I walked in, his daughter's face lit up with joyful recognition. "Daddy," she said choking back tears, "this is one of the doctors that saved your life."

It was truly a thrill to meet and again care for the man. The years of life that I was proud to have helped add allowed him to attend graduations, to celebrate birthdays and weddings, and to meet his first great-grandchild.

Had he died during that long ago night, it would have been a great disappointment. But time had caused me to forget most of the nameless faces and faceless names that filled the ceaseless days and sleepless nights of my residency. Having him for a patient became a source of great pride and he would always have a special place in my heart.

When he died peacefully in his sleep four years later, a part of me died with him.

Saving Lives

I saved a man's life today.

"Doctor," his wife exclaimed as she rushed though the office and embraced me, "I just had to stop by your office and thank you for all that you've done!"

"How is he?" I asked, somewhat startled by her excitement.

"Beautiful," she replied, "the surgeon said that he was amazed at how well he had come through the surgery. He expects him to be home in a few days."

"That's fantastic," I said. "He's a wonderful man. I'm sure he'll do fine."

Her husband was a fifty-eight year old accountant who had undergone surgery to repair an abdominal aortic aneurysm.

"The surgeon said it was over eight centimeters," she enthusiastically continued. "He said it was one of the biggest he had ever seen. He said that it could have ruptured at any moment. He was a walking time bomb. He said, 'you must have a great family doctor, he definitely saved your husband's life'. He was astonished that you picked up on it."

Her husband had come to see me for pain in his abdomen two weeks earlier. He had been in good health prior to his visit. He had smoked in the past, had borderline high blood pressure and was slightly overweight but had recently begun exercising and was feeling well. He had been drinking beer for a few days prior to his visit and had been taking ibuprofen for back pain. He was slightly tender in the area of his stomach but his exam was otherwise normal.

I sent him for an upper GI series and an ultrasound of his abdomen. The upper GI was normal but the ultrasound showed a large aneurysm. The radiologist was alarmed by the size and called me immediately. I was able to get him in to see a surgeon quickly and arrange to have it repaired.

"How long have we been your patients?" she asked.

"I don't know," I answered, "I guess six or seven years."

"I remember when we started coming," she gushed, still glowing with gratitude. "My sister referred us. She thought we would like you. I am so glad that we picked you for our doctor. I might be a widow if we hadn't."

She again hugged me and gave me a peck on the cheek. I was somewhat overwhelmed as I stood there proudly before her with my chin held high. She thought I was the greatest doctor in the world. I felt more like a fraud.

I thought he had had an ulcer. I did the upper GI to try to show it. I added an ultrasound just in case it might have been his gallbladder and because he was going to the radiologist anyway. An abdominal aortic aneurysm? The thought never even crossed my mind. He was at very low risk for this and his symptoms were certainly not that of an abdominal aneurysm. To this day I am certain that his abdominal pain came from the ibuprofen and having too much to drink

I accepted her gratitude with mixed emotions. I tried to rationalize it in my mind. Some of the world's greatest scientific discoveries were made by accident. I never heard anyone criticize Alexander Fleming for having discovered Penicillin by accident.

As much as I kicked the facts around in my head and in spite of his family thinking I was such a great doctor, I knew that I had arrived at his diagnosis completely by accident.

But none of that mattered. I saved a man's life today.

My Greatest Inspiration

I looked at the report with stunned silence. Young people are admitted to the hospital frequently for abdominal pain. The diagnoses are usually readily apparent. Appendicitis, gallstones, kidney stones or perhaps an ulcer came to mind.

But for this twenty-five year old man, none of those more obvious conditions seemed to be the case. His labs and X-rays were normal. He had been admitted during the night and this morning had an ultrasound of his abdomen. I read it in disbelief. There was a large mass in his abdomen. The report surmised that the mass might be arising from the pancreas or perhaps involving lymph nodes.

I scrutinized the report closely, trying to find a ray of optimism. But every plausible diagnosis I could think of was bad. The ultrasound could not determine a specific diagnosis, but some form of cancer was most likely. No matter how many times I examined the report, I could not deny the obvious. It was big, and it was there.

The next day, using a CT scan for guidance, the radiologist inserted a large needle into the young man's abdomen and biopsied the mass. Next came the waiting for the pathology report. It would be three interminable days.

Finally, on a Sunday morning the surgeon came in and sat down to talk to the young man. The young man's mother sat nervously by his side.

"Good morning!" the surgeon pleasantly said. The patient and his mother anxiously returned his greeting.

"We've gotten the biopsy back. Now, it is a tumor, but I'm having someone who specializes in this come in to see you and we're going to treat you as soon as possible."

"Is it cancer?" the patient's mother urgently questioned.

The surgeon turned slowly towards her. "Yes," he replied, "but we're going to treat it aggressively. He's in good hands. We're going to get through this."

The young man and his mother thanked the surgeon and he warmly shook their hands. They both remained stoically seated, trying to comprehend the magnitude of what had been told them.

I entered the same room. A dense gloom filled the air. Few words were spoken. I had seen patients receive, and have often been the bearer of such devastating news. I have always had trouble reading their faces. Was the quietness a sign of strength or a result of simply being overwhelmed?

I had always tried to be as compassionate as possible but it was truly difficult to understand what patients and their families were going through. For the one thing they all had in common was that they were always someone else. It was never me or my family.

In the months that followed, I walked with the young man through the valley of the shadow of death. I saw his ravaged body as he underwent surgeries and chemotherapy. I listened calmly as his oncologist told me that his cancer had spread to his lungs and his chance of survival was only about 15%. And I celebrated with him when he was still standing five years later.

The young man's journey helped me to understand the physical, emotional and spiritual struggles that a cancer patient and his family must endure. And more than any single event in my life, it helped me to be a more understanding and compassionate doctor.

It affected me not because of his young age, the severity of his illness nor the miracle of his survival. It affected me because he was my brother.

11

Family Ties

Ties that Bind

Within five minutes of entering the room, tears and sorrow replaced the smile and pleasantries that had greeted me. Two weeks prior to our visit, the young man's forty-seven year old father had died suddenly of a heart attack.

I had known the young man for three years and had never seen him so devastated. He had been very close to his father. He had worked with his father as an electrician for the past six years.

The young man was twenty-eight years old, had been married for five years and had a two-year-old son who was snuggled closely on his father's lap. He tearfully talked about the closeness of his family. He had spent every day working with his father and many evenings at his parent's house with his wife and son.

As I consoled my patient, my mind kept returning to an unsettling thought. My patient's father was overweight and suffered from diabetes, high cholesterol and high blood pressure. Most men in the family died before reaching fifty.

As my patient was talking, I glanced down at his chart. At twenty-eight, he was already on medication for high blood pressure and high cholesterol. He had gained thirty pounds since getting married and his blood sugars were borderline high. To make matters even worse, he smoked a pack of cigarettes a day.

"Do you take after your father?" I asked.

My question brought a smile to his face. "Everyone says I have my father's eyes," he replied.

He did have distinctive deep blue eyes that stood out in contrast to his fair complexion and light red hair and strongly resembled those of his father's.

"I know what you're getting at, Doc," he continued, "my father lost his father when he was about my age. Now my dad is gone. I know I have to start taking better care of myself so I'm around for my kids."

I was pleased that he had gotten my point. Perhaps he could give up smoking, lose weight, and begin to exercise and eat right. Perhaps he could be the first man in his family to collect social security. Yet I knew that bad genes could be hard to overcome.

My heart broke for the young man's misfortune. Not only for having lost his father, his son's grandfather, at such a young age but also for his own already poor health. He was a hostage to the genetics that had passed through his family for generations, had killed his father and would likely someday kill him. Even more, I felt sorry for his two-year-old son, the next generation who sat quietly on his father's lap, staring at me suspiciously with his deep blue eyes.

Mexican Cancer Treatment

As I sat listening to her, my mind was searching for the right words to say. She had come seeking my advice, yet I knew it was the last thing she wanted to hear.

She was a lovely twenty-four year old woman. Two years ago she graduated college. And she had to grow up in a hurry.

The summer after her college graduation, she returned home to live with her divorced mother and sixteen year old brother. She brought her forty-eight year old mother to her doctor to evaluate her fatigue and abdominal bloating. He evaluated her and quickly found the source of her problem. Their lives would never be the same. Her mother had a cancerous tumor growing from her left ovary.

They proceeded along the standard course of treatment. She had surgery to remove the cancer and followed with chemotherapy. She did well for a while, but within a year the cancer was back. Further treatment slowed the progression of the disease but was unable to cure her.

"I was looking for information on the Internet," she began, "and I found out about this cancer treatment center in Mexico. They use high doses of intravenous vitamins to boost the patient's immune system so their own immune system can rid their bodies of cancer."

I was immediately suspicious. "Did they tell you how effective the treatment was?" I asked.

"Yes," she answered, "I spoke to a doctor there and he told me that about ninety-five percent of the patients are cured."

"Ninety-five percent were cured?" I questioned. "Then why isn't the treatment available in the United States?"

"I think he said they were cured," she answered. "The reason he said it wasn't available in the United States was that it is so cheap. He said drug companies make so much money treating cancer that they're able to keep high dose vitamins from being FDA approved."

"How expensive is the treatment?" I asked.

"Well, we'll have to fly to Mexico and stay there," she answered, "and every day go to the clinic to receive the treatment. It's just vitamins, nothing toxic, so my mom will feel okay. We'll be down there for two weeks and with the flight and motel I expect to spend somewhere between ten and fifteen thousand."

I was immediately suspicious. My stomach turned as I thought of the clinic, free of American laws, stealing the life savings of desperate families in exchange for false hope.

But as I looked her in the eyes, they filled with the fire of hope that I knew I could not extinguish. I explained to her some of my suspicions, but wished her the best of luck.

Perhaps it was the vitamins, perhaps the warm Mexican climate, but her mother felt well during those two weeks. It turned out to be a wonderful trip. The treatment left time for long walks on the beach, quiet dinners and long talks in their motel room. It was a time of joy and hope, free from the pessimism of her American doctors.

It was a time the young woman would always treasure and never forget. The memories would fill her heart and sustain her love, especially three months later when her mother passed away.

Time Enough for Peace

As I drove towards his house for what I feared would be the last time, my mind wandered back to a conversation we had had a few short years ago.

He had sat bravely before me, a handsome, out-going thirty-three year old accountant. We talked about his job and his recent vacation. We talked about the weather and the World Series. We talked about his latest CD4 counts and how he was tolerating his daily drug cocktail that was controlling his AIDS infection.

The conversation was, as always, upbeat. But his mood changed as the conversation moved to his parents.

"I'll never forget what happened when I was a kid," he said as he sadly shook his head, "I got into trouble at school and was terrified that my parents would find out."

"My teacher called that night," he slowly continued, "I can still remember my parents coming into my room to talk to me. They were so disappointed, not because I got into trouble but because I didn't come to them. I'll never forget my father's words. 'We're your parents,' he pleaded with me, 'you can tell us anything. No matter what ever happens in your life you can come to us and we'll be there for you.'"

"If I robbed a bank, if I killed someone . . . I guess they would have been okay, but when I finally got up the courage to tell them . . . to tell them I was gay," he hesitantly continued, "they disowned me. They stopped calling me. They barely would look at me. I just stopped trying."

As his disease progressed, the pain deepened. After years of doing well, he was diagnosed with non-Hodgkin's lymphoma and his health declined rapidly.

He had known that his remaining days were now few and as I walked to his door I wondered if his parents were even aware.

When I knocked at his door, an older woman answered. She had tired eyes, tousled hair and a worried expression. When I told her who I was, she smiled, wiped her hands on her apron and reached out to shake my hand.

"Thank you for coming," she replied, "I'm his mother, come right this way."

As I entered his room, he was lying in a hospital bed. His skin was pale and clammy and his body had wasted away to almost nothing. He forced a smile as I gently squeezed his hand.

By his bed sat his father. He was a large and powerful appearing man who appeared to be in his sixties. As he smiled at me I could see he had been crying. He carefully lifted his son from the bed so I could listen to his lungs and lovingly fluffed his pillow as he lowered his head back down. Later, as I wrote a note in his chart, his father softly wiped his forehead with a cool towel then gently placed a kiss.

The loving care of his parents had softened the horror of a dying young man that I had prepared myself to witness.

I found out later that a friend of the young man had contacted his parents. The years had caused them to regret the way they had treated their son and when they found out he was dying they rushed to his side.

He nodded and smiled weakly as I left and I knew that the end was near. There would never be time to make up for all the lost moments they had never shared. There would never be time to resolve all the words and emotions that had passed between them through the years.

But as I looked at the contentment on his face, I knew that there was time enough to find peace.

The Secret

"Doesn't mom look great!" he nearly shouted before I had even entered the room.

I looked down at her thin, frail body as she lay silently in her hospital bed. Her eyes were sunken, her skin a pasty yellow and her lips were parched and cracked. My mind screamed "No", but my words hesitantly spoke, "Yes, she's coming along real well."

But his mother did not look well. She looked like a woman in the final stages of a battle with cancer who was ready to go home and die. She had been a robust woman who was now failing rapidly.

"Yeah, she's really doing great," her son continued, "she's eating well and slowly building her strength. We'll have her up and around in no time."

She smiled weakly towards me. Her untouched lunch tray sat ominously before her. She looked like she was dying of cancer because she was in fact at the end of a long courageous battle against colon cancer.

As I examined her, I was unable to find a ray of hope that would support her son's optimism. Her eyes and skin were yellow. There was fluid in her lungs, her abdomen was distended and her legs were grossly swollen.

I told her she was ready to go home and that I would fill out her discharge paperwork. As I walked towards the nurses' station, her son quickly followed me.

"Mom's not a very strong person," he implored, "she couldn't bear the thought of dying. I know my mom better than anyone and I'm sure she can't handle knowing the truth. I didn't tell her that the visiting nurse is a hospice nurse. She thinks she is just going home to build up her strength so she can get surgery or chemo."

"I don't agree with you," I replied, "I think your mother has been very strong throughout this whole ordeal and I'd like to be straightforward with her."

"Please don't tell her, Doc," he pleaded, "it would destroy her to know she was dying. She can't handle it. Trust me, I know my mom."

With reservations, I finally agreed to play along with his charade but I refused to lie if she asked me any direct questions about her condition. This made me feel better, but I knew there would be no such questions.

My mind raced as I slowly walked back down the corridor towards her room. I wondered how she could not realize how sick she was. I resented her son for not having the courage to deal honestly with the situation. But most of all I was angry with myself for letting her son pressure me into compromising our doctor-patient relationship

She was alone when I returned to her room to give her the discharge papers and her prescriptions. I explained the instructions to her. She weakly reached towards me and I held her hand.

"Take care of yourself," I told her.

"Thank you for everything you've done for me and for my family," she said with an air of finality, "you've been a great help. I thank God I have my son to take care of me. I don't know what I would do without him."

I nodded in agreement as she continued to hold my hand.

"This is hard for him," she said, "when his father died a few years ago he really had a hard time. He couldn't even talk about it. You understand."

She released my hand and patted me reassuringly on the arm. "Thank you for not telling my son that I'm dying."

Remembering Uncle Pete

"Does your son play baseball?" she asked as I stood up to examine her husband.

"Yes," I answered, "he does. Why do you ask?"

"Oh, I think I saw him," she explained, "I was in the store a few weeks ago and I think I saw him."

I walked over to her husband as he sat silently on the examining table. I smiled at him and he smiled softly back. He was an eighty-three year old man who looked much younger. He had a full head of gray hair, a warm smile and was well groomed and dressed. He would always sport a golf shirt and looked like he had just stepped off a Palm Beach golf course. He had a few wrinkles that appeared when he smiled although his smile had become less frequent in recent years. I remembered when he had an animated personality, a witty sense of humor and an active social life that included frequent rounds of golf, dining and traveling with his wife. Conversation now was mostly short questions and one word answers.

"How did you know it was my son?" I asked his wife as I began my examination.

"I saw MARZILI written on the back of his baseball uniform," she explained. "It's not a very common name so I figured it was your son."

I nodded as I held my stethoscope against her husband's chest.

"Take a deep breath," I said. He had always been able to follow my simple commands but this time did nothing. "Take a deep breath," I repeated. Still nothing.

Finally, after a long pause, he spoke. "Is there a Pete Marzili?"

His question took me by surprise. His wife and I looked at each other with puzzled expressions. A fog seemed to have had lifted from his mind as he looked at me inquisitively.

"I had an Uncle Pete," I curiously answered, "he was Pete Marzili."

After another pause he continued, "We served in the Army together. We trained together. I knew him."

He was my father's oldest brother. Long before I was born he had settled near Dallas, Texas to work and raise his family. I had met him but a few times and remember him only as a middle-aged man with grown children. I knew he had served in the Army during World War II. I remember seeing a picture of him in his Army uniform at my grandmother's house many years ago. I never thought much about it as a child but now became curious about this chance glimpse into my family's past. I knew the opportunity would be fleeting.

"Did you serve together long?" I pressed, "Did you know him well?"

He again appeared confused. "No," he slowly answered, "no. We shipped out together but when we got to Europe we were separated and ended up in different outfits. We lost touch. He was a nice fellow."

I struggled to imagine them as young soldiers, just boys really, on their way to the great crusade against tyranny in Europe. They bravely survived everything Hitler and the German war machine could throw at them and returned home safely to humbly live their lives. Curiously, it would be a kindly German doctor named Alois Alzheimer that would describe the disease that would eventually devastate both of their lives.

"He died about five years ago," I said although no one had asked. I stopped myself before saying that he had died in a nursing home of Alzheimer's disease. I do not recall feeling any great sorrow when I had learned of this distant uncle's death. As I sat there talking about him with his old army buddy, I felt a closeness to my uncle that I had never known and the sadness of his death felt more significant. His loss more personal.

"You knew my uncle a long time ago," I said, "I'm very impressed that you remembered him."

I was afraid that I had sounded patronizing. It did not matter as he was again lost in his silent stare.

I wanted to ask more. I hoped to learn more about my uncle's experiences during the war. About his family. About my family. I would always gratefully treasure the gift of these long lost memories of an uncle that I barely had the opportunity to know. But as I peered deeply into his eyes I could see that the window of opportunity had closed and I wondered if it would ever open again.

A Great Time to be Alive

"I see you're retired," I said as I reviewed his medical history form, "what are you retired from?"

"Engineering," he replied, "but I did just about everything. I used to play ball for the Red Sox. Well, I never actually made the big leagues, you see, but I spent a few seasons pitching for their farm teams. I went to Spring Training one year with a fellow named Ted Williams. I once pitched to Babe Ruth. It was at the end of his career but I'll bet that you never met anyone who pitched to Babe Ruth."

He smiled and ran his large fingers through his thick gray hair. He was a delightful elderly gentleman who had recently moved to the area to be near his daughter. He stood over me at about six foot three and still looked like he could play baseball in spite of a cane that lent an air of distinction rather than disability.

"That really must have been something," I said.

"Yeah," he shrugged, "I loved baseball. I thought I could make the big leagues. But it was the Depression and there wasn't much money in baseball. One off-season I met this great girl. I was crazy about her. We fell in love and wanted to get married so I needed a steady job. Her dad worked in the shipyard and got me a job. I've got no regrets about quitting baseball. It was a tough way to make a living in those days. War came a couple of years later so I would have been drafted anyway. Never pitched a day in the big leagues but was married to my beautiful bride for sixty wonderful years."

"She died?" I asked.

"Yep," he replied, "she died of heart failure three years ago. But we had a great life together."

"So you made a career out of the shipyard?" I asked.

"Could have," he answered, "had a deferment from the military because of my job at the shipyard. But I enlisted anyway. Fought my way across Italy and France. Still got some shrapnel in my butt. Souvenir from Monte Cassino. We were training to invade Japan when they dropped the bomb. Hard for people to understand today but that was the happiest day of my life. Not many of us figured on coming home before that. After the war I took advantage of the GI bill and got a degree in engineering. Then I went back to the shipyard."

"You've had quite an interesting life," I commented.

"I've seen a lot of history," he humbly replied, "a lot of history."

I looked at him in admiration as he described his life. He had witnessed and taken part in some of the most significant events of the past century. As he neared the end of his life, I could not help but think how lucky he was to have lived during this time. I continued through his medical history form but I paused as I looked at his family history.

"You wrote that your mother and two of your sisters died of influenza," I questioned, thinking it was a mistake.

"That's right, they all died of the same disease," he answered in a slow drawl, "the same day."

My startled face prompted him to continue.

"I was just two years old so I don't remember much," he said as he slowly shook his head, "it was during the influenza epidemic of 1918. Hit our family hard. Hit a lot of families hard. My eight year old sister died in the morning. My mom was pregn ant and real sick. She delivered the baby that afternoon but died shortly after. The baby died later that night."

I had read that a staggering 675,000 Americans died in that tragic epidemic of 1918 but had never fully appreciated the human impact.

He smiled and patted me reassuringly on the shoulder. "It's a great time to be alive," he said.

At first I thought he was talking about his own life. But then I realized he was talking about mine.

12

Broken Hearts

Unforgettable

I have a picture in my mind of a freckled face and braces on her teeth. Her strawberry blonde hair in pigtails hanging from under a baseball cap. It was long ago on a Saturday morning and she had been hit in the head during a softball game. Perhaps it was the first time I ever saw her. I remember her grin and I knew that she would be okay.

At intervals of time I would see her. The sports physicals and forms for summer camp. The ear infections, poison ivy and sprained ankles. Sometimes every two months. Sometimes every year. I would ask her about school and sports and her friends. I looked upon her with wonder as she changed so much on each encounter and watched her mature into a lovely young lady.

She was not the captain of the cheerleaders. Nor did her grades earn her a spot on the honor roll. She did not star on the soccer team. She was not elected homecoming queen.

She was a decent student in high school, earning mostly B's and C's. She was on the soccer team but was rarely given the opportunity to play. She had a boyfriend and a small group of close friends.

She never got into trouble. She rarely missed school. She did not smoke or use drugs. She never touched alcohol. She did not get pregnant. She had a great relationship with her parents and younger brother.

She was like the majority of high school students who pass through their schools without earning great accolades and without being remembered for the trouble they caused. The kind of kid who did nothing to distinguish herself from her classmates yet of whom any parent would be proud.

Her visits with me were not particularly memorable and my recollections of our encounters have largely faded. Her mother or father would usually bring her when she was little. She was a shy young girl and would sit quietly as I examined her.

When she was older and could drive she would come alone but less frequent. She was becoming more independent and was easier to talk to. She would occasionally bring her little brother for his office visits and was a responsible older sister.

She was developing into a very nice young woman. She was the type of woman who would go to college or perhaps get a job. She would fall in love and get married. She would buy a house and have children.

As time passes, my memories of her become more obscure. Though I now try, I can scarcely remember her face.

The last time I saw her was more than two years ago. Still, I think of her every day. For as I drive home to my family at the end of the day I pass a tree by a curve on the road. By that tree there is a pile of faded cards and lovingly placed flowers that surround a simple wooden cross that bears her name.

Dear Doctor

I looked at the form with surprise and hurt. It was a simple form, the medical equivalent of a Dear John letter. A patient who I thought I had a good relationship with was requesting that I transfer his medical records to another family physician.

Was he moving? No. The new doctor was nearby. He just wanted a different physician.

I had met him two years ago when he had come in with his wife. She was only forty-nine years old but was a very sick woman. She had not been to the doctor in years but had decided to come in when a "cold" had lasted for over a month.

She had smoked a pack of cigarettes a day for over thirty years but had quit two weeks prior. Her coarse, hacking cough had become progressively worse and for the previous two days she had been coughing up blood. She had lost fifteen pounds over the past two months and had an emaciated appearance.

I took no satisfaction in my ability to diagnose her. It was as straightforward as medicine can get. The woman had lung cancer. I had hoped that maybe it was a bad case of pneumonia but a chest X-ray quickly proved otherwise.

I clearly remember when they came back to my office the following day to review the chest X-ray. They both could see the writing on the wall but were still unable to prepare themselves for what I had to tell them.

"How are you?" I asked.

"A little better," she answered, "what did the X-ray show?"

"It did show what appears to be a mass in your left lung," I began to explain.

She became unsteady in her seat and held her husband for support. I did my best to be compassionate and optimistic. I went on to explain the situation and likely treatment but I was sure that neither one of them heard another word.

I saw them sporadically as she went through her treatments. There was little hope of curing her but she responded well to radiation therapy and enjoyed a decent quality of life for the next year.

I sadly remember one of the last times I saw her. Her fight for life was becoming increasingly difficult. Her quality of life had become so poor that she no longer wanted to continue the struggle. It was an emotional and tearful moment when she accepted the inevitability of her death and we began to make arrangements for hospice care.

After her death, her husband sent me a touching card thanking me for all that I had done. The card made it even harder to understand why he was now leaving.

Months later, I finally found out why he had transferred. He was not dissatisfied with my medical treatment. He was not unhappy with the way I cared for his family during the most difficult time in their lives.

Had I known him longer, perhaps he would have felt differently. But when he came into my office, it would evoke the memories of a time of unspeakable sorrow. At a time when he was striving to remember the good times, a visit to my office would make him recall the worst of times. All the care that I had given him and for which he would be forever grateful no longer mattered. For it happened in my office, and I would always be the doctor who told him his wife had cancer.

A Lesson in Life

It was a dreary Sunday morning as I entered the Intensive Care Unit. Her age and appearance seemed out of place compared to the critically ill patients that usually dwell there.

She was an attractive, healthy appearing seventeen year old girl. Her long brown hair was neatly pulled back in a ponytail and she was reclining comfortably in her bed. Her TV was playing and a magazine was on her lap as she chatted happily on the phone. Cards and flowers neatly lined the window sill. Only the activated charcoal draining from her nasogastric tube hinted to the reason for her being there.

I had known her family since I had started in practice. She was a popular girl and a good student who was planning to go to college next year. The night she was admitted her boyfriend broke up with her. She came home upset and had a fight with her parents. Thinking her life was not worth living, she decided to end it by taking a bottle of pills.

"When can I go home?" she asked the moment I approached, "I'm going crazy in here and I have a lot of homework to do."

I sat down beside her bed and began perusing her chart. She was medically stable. The psychiatrist had evaluated her and believed she no longer posed a threat to herself.

As we talked, she expressed regret for what she had done and felt stupid for having done it. Still, I was not convinced that she realized how close she had come to dying and the devastating affect her suicide attempt had had on her family.

As I began completing her discharge forms, I noticed her staring across the ICU at another patient.

"Does he have cancer?" she asked.

I looked across the ICU at a very ill appearing young man lying in the bed. His thin pale body lay motionless except for the rising and falling of his chest with each pump of the ventilator. His mother sat bravely beside him lovingly caressing his arm while other family members stood helplessly by.

"Yes," I answered.

I was also surprised to see another young patient in the ICU that day. He was not my patient but I was familiar with his story. He was stricken two years ago with a rare and aggressive cancer called Ewing's sarcoma. He bravely persevered months of chemotherapy. Unfortunately, his cancer was discovered too late and proved unstoppable. He had not yet given up the fight and was still being treated aggressively and battling tenaciously for life.

"How old is he?" she asked.

"Seventeen," I replied, "your age."

"Is he going to die?" she asked.

"I don't know," I answered as I looked up at his chest X-ray hanging ominously outside his room and showing several large tumors that had spread to his lungs. "It doesn't look very hopeful."

As I got up to leave, her eyes and attention remained fixated on the young man who fought on against insurmountable odds to preserve the difficult life he held so sacred. I was struck by the irony of her willingness to throw away her own precious life.

I started to speak but the words froze in my throat. But as I looked into her eyes, I knew that there was nothing my words could add to what she had already learned from the dying young man whom she would never have the opportunity to know.

How Did He Die?

"How did he die," she asked as she stoically wiped her tears.

I looked into her eyes and studied her face as I tried to measure how much information she really wanted.

"Well," I tentatively replied, "we had talked before about his heart condition and how severely damaged his heart was."

"He had another heart attack?" she asked.

"No, he didn't have another heart attack," I answered, realizing that even at this moment she would not let me escape without a more detailed answer.

"His heart was severely damaged from his last heart attack," I continued, "and he had congestive heart failure. His heart just couldn't pump the blood well enough and the fluid kept backing up into his lungs. That's why he often became so short of breath and why his legs kept swelling."

She continued to listen to me intently although I was not sure how much she was comprehending.

"Didn't the medicine work?" she asked.

"The medicine did work," I replied, "it undoubtedly let him enjoy his life for a few extra years. But it couldn't change the damage that was already done."

She trembled slightly as she tried to grasp what I was telling her.

"Believe me," I added, "I know what was done to your husband and if it gives you any comfort I can assure you that everything possible was done to save his life."

She seemed reassured as she smiled slightly, hugged me and thanked me for all I had done.

"Oh, doctor," she called as I turned to leave, "did he suffer?"

I froze in my tracks as the words reverberated in my mind. I remembered the terror in his eyes as he looked into the worried faces of the doctors and nurses as they rushed him down the hall to the ICU.

I recalled how he fought desperately as the intubation tube was placed down his throat. Despite heavy sedation, he continued to thrash violently until he was able to pull the tube out. I saw the anger in his face as his arms were restrained to the side rails so the tube could be replaced and watched him wince in pain and struggle to pull away as the respiratory therapist penetrated his radial artery to obtain an arterial blood gas.

When I had examined him, his eyes pleaded with me to stop the suffering. I had patted him on the shoulder to reassure him as I turned away. I could feel his eyes piercing me as I walked from his bed and could not bring myself to look back at him.

He needed stronger doses of sedation to finally calm his agitation before he finally was able to sleep.

I remembered hearing "Code Blue, ICU" resonate through the hospital corridors and I knew that it was him. His body jolted violently from the bed with each shock from the defibrillator as the medical staff worked aggressively to save him. But it soon became apparent that his body had had enough.

I would have done anything to have made him more comfortable, but now I could only hope to bring some measure of comfort to his wife.

I hesitantly looked back into her sorrowful, waiting eyes.

"No," I answered, "he died peacefully."

Empty Life

I drove hurriedly to his house but hesitated as I approached the door. I did not know what I would find. He was a hospice patient in the terminal stages of liver cancer. I knew that he was near death and wanted to see him before he died. I had called several times that day but had gotten no answer.

His sister-in-law greeted me at the door with a sorrowful look in her eye. I introduced myself and told her I had been trying to call all day.

"Sorry," she shrugged, "we knew that the end was near so we left the phone off the hook."

"How is he doing?" I asked.

"Breathing real shallow," she answered, "I don't think he has very long."

There were mixed emotions in her voice. He was her sister's husband and I sensed she did not have a high opinion of him. He usually came to see me in the morning and always seemed pleasant. But I knew things changed once he started drinking. And he drank every day. I often smelled the alcohol on his breath at nine in the morning. He would drink at least two six-packs of beer a day and often some scotch or vodka.

His wife stayed with him but her resentment towards him increased over the years. He was verbally abusive towards her and I had always suspected he may have been physically abusive but she would never admit to it.

His sister-in-law led me to his room then turned her back and walked away. His wife got up from her bedside chair, walked over and hugged me. His twenty-four year old daughter sat curled up in a chair, sobbing in the corner of the room. His twenty-two year old son was dressed in camouflage, his head was shaven and he was anxiously pacing the floor.

The room was dark except for the late afternoon sunlight that squeezed through the partially closed blinds. An empty beer can sat on the nightstand. I had tried to get him to stop drinking but eventually realized that it no longer mattered.

He lay silently on the bed. He was gaunt, yellow, his eyes were wide open, his mouth gaping, and there were no signs of breathing. I bent over him and reached down with my stethoscope to listen for his heart. After a few moments, I stood up and almost bumped into his son who was standing over me. His face was about 12 inches from mine and he had a wild look in his eyes.

"Is he . . ." he asked, then took his finger like a knife and made a slicing motion across his throat. It was the strangest way someone had ever asked me if a loved one had died and it will always stick in my mind.

"Yes," I answered, "I'm very sorry."

His daughter cried a bit louder and his wife walked slowly towards his bed.

"So I guess that's it, then," she said in a tired voice.

"Is there anything I can do?" I asked.

"No," she answered, "I'm alright. Do you have to sign something?"

"Not now," I replied, "the funeral director will drop off the death certificate."

When I left that afternoon, I felt a strange but deep sadness. There is a beauty in death that comes from the outpouring of love and marks the end of a full and wonderful life. There was no beauty in that room that day. The sadness that I felt was not so much for the sorrow of his death, but for the emptiness that was his life.

13

Divine Intervention

Prayer for a Patient

I sat bolt upright in the church pew and a chill ran down my spine as her name was read among the sick of the parish for whom the church would pray. Most of the people whose names were read were strangers to me, but her I knew well. The distress of attending to a suffering patient had disturbed my tranquility at church.

She was a wonderful and healthy seventy year old woman who had a zest for life. I had known her for the past five years and would see her in the office every three or four months for her high blood pressure or an occasional cold. Much more frequently I would say hello or share a conversation after church.

Two years ago she saw me for pain in her right upper abdomen. I examined her and sent her for an ultrasound that showed several small gallstones. I referred her to a surgeon who recommended removing her gallbladder.

Over the next few days the pain lessened. She was not the type of person who would take medications or have tests done unless they were absolutely necessary. When her abdominal pain resolved, she decided not to proceed with the surgery.

"I'm not going to let them cut me as long as I'm feeling good," she said, "I'll just watch my diet and see if I can treat this myself."

We discussed the pros and cons of her decision and agreed that she would watch her fat intake and see me right away if the pain returned.

She did well for the next two years and had no further pain. Then her pain returned with a vengeance. The amount of pain was disconcerting. Her right upper abdomen was extremely tender and she had a jaundiced appearance. I immediately sent her to the surgeon who at once took her to the operating room to remove her gallbladder.

What he found was her gallbladder with stones but not causing any problems. The source of her pain was not her gallbladder but several tumors that had spread from a previously unknown ovarian cancer and were now obstructing her liver.

Ahead of her lay perhaps radiation or chemotherapy. Perhaps only death.

To most of the people in the church she was a stranger. I knew her well, yet the familiarity we shared could bring me little solace. I was her doctor but as I looked around the crowded church I knew that I could do little more for her than anyone else in the church.

As a doctor, sometimes we can heal a patient by writing a prescription, performing a procedure, or referring them to an appropriate specialist. Sometimes we can reach for the stars and from the deepest recesses of our mind retrieve a long forgotten diagnosis or treatment and look like the greatest doctor in the world. These things all seemed to have little relevance now as I sat tormented by my inability to treat her.

So as the choir sang and the sun danced through the stained glass window, I did the only thing I could. I bowed my head and prayed.

God's Will

"You look fantastic," I told her, "I can't believe you just had surgery three weeks ago."

"Thank you," she said with a broad smile, "everyone tells me I'm doing great!"

"And when are you going to be seeing the oncologist again?" I asked.

"No more," she proudly answered, "I'm all cured. Praise the Lord!"

I wanted to congratulate her and share in her joy but was confused about the facts of her case. I rapidly began fumbling through her chart. She had come in to see me six weeks earlier complaining of fatigue and shortness of breath. She was found to be very anemic and losing blood through her intestinal track. I sent her to a gastroenterologist who promptly performed a colonoscopy and found a cancerous tumor in her colon.

I pulled out the letter from the surgeon, which reaffirmed my memory that when the tumor was removed, it was found to have spread to her lymph nodes. How could she not have known this?

"Um," I stuttered, hating to burst her bubble, "didn't the doctor mention that they found the cancer in your lymph nodes?"

"Oh, yes," she replied, still full of enthusiasm, "but he still thought I was cured."

"Sure," I said, "but they usually recommend chemotherapy when the tumor spreads to your lymph nodes. There is no guarantee either way but your chances are much better with the chemo."

"He told me the same thing," she answered, "but I don't think I need it. I have complete faith that the Lord has healed me. I prayed to Jesus and I feel His power in me."

I had the greatest respect for her faith but fought with all my heart to change her mind.

"Cancer treatments have been studied extensively," I explained. "If you get the chemotherapy, it will improve your chances of a cure. It will improve your chances of not dying."

She looked at me sternly. "I don't need to improve my chances of a cure. I am cured." And that was the final word.

On a winter's afternoon sixteen months later, she sat in the same room waiting for me. I had seen her that morning for abdominal pain and nausea. She had an ill appearance and the whites of her eyes were yellow. I had sent her for an abdominal ultrasound and some labs and told her to return that afternoon.

I studied the test results as I summoned the strength to break the news to her. I entered the room to find her sitting passively in the chair. She already knew.

"What do the tests show?" she asked.

"I'm sorry," I answered, "but the ultrasound revealed a number of masses in your liver."

"The cancer spread?" she calmly asked.

"That's what it looks like," I replied, "I'm very sorry."

"It's okay," she calmly said, forcing a smile, "I guess that's the Lord's will."

From the time I had seen her months earlier, I had hoped and prayed that her story would have a different ending. But that was not how it happened. I firmly believe in the healing and comforting power of prayer but I have also witnessed the life saving miracle of modern medicine. I will always wonder if God had sent the answer to her prayers and she had just failed to recognize it.

Doubting Miracles

"It happened so quickly," she said, "one minute he was riding his bike up and down the driveway waving at us, the next minute he was lying in the street unconscious."

She had been visiting her daughter on a perfect spring day. But the beauty of the day was instantly and forever shattered by the screeching of a car's brakes and the unforgettable sound of the car striking her four year old grandson. She was tearfully telling me about her grandson who at that moment was in a coma, fighting for his life. I had never met her grandson but felt I knew him well. He was her first and only grandchild and she relished showing his pictures and telling stories about him.

She had a wonderful life. She had a loving husband with whom she traveled the world. Every time I saw her she was returning from or about to leave on an exotic vacation or just enjoying the tranquility of her house at the beach. She had a close relationship with her daughter and loved to spend time with her grandson.

But in one tragic moment, her entire life had changed.

She looked me in the eyes. Her tears stopped flowing. The sadness on her face melted away into anger.

"How could he let this happen?" she nearly shouted, "He's only four years old."

"How could who let it happen?" I inquired.

"God!" she furiously stated, then paused to compose herself. "God, I mean if there even is a God, how could he let this happen? He's only four years old. What kind of horrible sin could he have committed to deserve such a horrible punishment? He's just a baby, just an innocent baby."

I had known her for years and had never seen such anger on her face. I had also never known her to be a religious person. Yet at this tragic time, she seemed to be focusing all of her energy into a deep rage against God.

"All my daughter wants is for everyone to pray for him, she thinks that will cure him," she said with a roll of her eyes, "I do it for her sake but its very difficult to pray to a God who would let something like this happen."

Her grandson's prognosis was poor and the doctors, while trying to be optimistic, prepared the family for the worst. For the next week he remained in a coma. As the rest of his family hoped and prayed for his recovery, I sensed that his grandmother was losing hope. She was inconsolable and began talking about him in the past tense.

Ten days after the accident, the miracle finally happened. The doctors were astounded when he not only awoke from his coma but within days was running the halls and appeared to suffer no permanent neurological damage.

When I saw the child's grandmother again, she was ecstatic. Her cherished grandson, who came precariously close to death, was well again. She raved about the skill of the wonderful doctors and the loving care of the devoted nurses and hospital staff.

Her life had miraculously returned to normal. She was again enjoying her grandson and anticipating a fun filled summer at the beach. She had just returned from a trip to West Palm Beach and was planning a summer Mediterranean cruise. Life was great. Everything was perfect again.

And that was the last I heard about God.

Angels

The wailing of the young mother pierced the monotonous droning of the monitors as I slowly walked through the Neonatal Intensive Care Unit during the wee hours of the morning. As a fourth-year medical student, I kept silent as the resident exchanged greetings with the hysterical mother and began to look at her listless newborn.

The mother did not speak English, so the resident enlisted the help of a Spanish speaking cleaning woman to help with translation. The cleaning woman did not speak English very well and had great difficulty with medical terms. But she was all we had.

Through her broken English, we were able to obtain the information we needed. The mother was twenty-three years old and this was her second pregnancy. Her first pregnancy ended in a miscarriage and she received no prenatal care for this pregnancy. She showed up in the emergency room the night before and delivered the baby. I was surprised at her strength as she sat there, having delivered the baby only hours earlier.

It was obvious to everyone that there was something seriously wrong with her baby. The baby barely moved except for an occasional brief seizure. His body appeared normal with ten little fingers, ten little toes and a puffy red face. But the entire top of his head was missing and his small and misshapen brain was grotesquely visible. The mother cried endlessly, which made the situation even more heart wrenching. We offered a few words of encouragement that she did not understand and we did not believe. We stood around awkwardly waiting for the Neonatologist to arrive.

Finally, he appeared. He had not been happy to have been awakened so early, but seemed genuinely excited about the interesting case. And eager to use his Spanish.

"Buenos diaz," he greeted the mother. Good morning.

She quietly returned his greeting as she wiped the tears from her eyes. "Que tiene de malo mi bebe?" She asked. What is wrong with my baby?

"El tiene . . . uh . . . anencephaly," he hesitantly answered. He has anencephaly.

"Que es eso?" she quickly asked. What is that?

He enthusiastically began to explain this rare and complicated syndrome when she abruptly interrupted. "Que se puede hacer?" What can be done?

His face dropped and his shoulders sagged. "Nada," he answered. Nothing.

She cried hysterically and inconsolably as we stood there helplessly.

"Lo siento," he said. I'm sorry. He then disconnected the monitors, wrapped the newborn's head with a blanket and gently placed the dying baby in his mother's arms.

She resumed her hysterical crying. We all stood there not knowing what to do. To walk away would have seemed heartless, but it felt even worse to stay. It seemed there was nothing anyone could do.

Then I saw her. She was walking intently towards us with a small bottle in her hand. The dawn was breaking and the sun's early morning rays shone upon her. We stood in silence as she knelt down beside the young mother. She opened the bottle and poured its water onto the baby's tiny head.

"Yo te bautizo," she said, "enel nombre del Padre, del Hijo, y del Espiritu Santo." Then she drew a cross on the baby's forehead and baptized him in the name of Father, the Son, and the Holy Spirit.

The mother's cries softened to a peaceful whimper. The neonatologist walked away to return to his office. The resident and I quietly moved to the next baby to begin our morning rounds. And the angel who had baptized the baby and brought such comfort to the grieving young mother, picked up her mop and went back to cleaning the floor.

14

Hope

The Last Brave Surgeon

"What's going to happen to me?" he asked, "the lung doctor says I'm not in good enough shape to be operated on. What chance do I have of beating lung cancer if they don't operate?"

If the question had appeared on a medical board exam it would have been quite simple: A sixty year old male who had smoked two packs of cigarettes a day for forty years and who suffers from emphysema presents with an inoperable three centimeter tumor of his left lung. What are his chances of being cured?

If it were a test question it would have been easy. But it was not a test question. It was a question posed by a dear patient of mine who was facing a life or death crisis.

"There are still a number of options," I answered, "radiation therapy is very effective at shrinking the tumor. Chemotherapy is also sometimes used."

"Yeah," he doubtfully replied, "but I'll still die. I just wish they could get the cancer out. I want a chance of being cured. They say I might die on the operating table but I'm willing to take that risk."

"The doctors in the hospital told you that they couldn't operate?" I asked.

"Well, the cardiologist thought my heart could take it," he answered, "but the lung doctor said my lungs couldn't handle it and the surgeon said he wouldn't touch me. It's ridiculous. They basically tell me I'm going to die anyway but they won't operate because they're afraid I'm going to die."

I sympathized with his argument. I thought his lungs were much improved since his hospitalization so I sent him for second opinions to a different lung specialist and a different surgeon. I did it for the reasons he had given but still had my own doubts.

To my surprise, he was cleared for surgery and the surgeon agreed to operate. Privately I wondered what the surgeon was thinking. From the size and location of the tumor, even if he survived the surgery it was likely that the cancer had already spread and his long-term prognosis was still statistically very poor. But the worst nightmare for the surgeon would be to have the patient die on the operating table. I knew that the surgeon was giving the patient his only hope for a cure. But I could also imagine the facts of the case being twisted by a sharp malpractice lawyer.

"Doctor," the lawyer could contend, "you operated on this patient knowing full well that he would probably not survive. The first lung specialist absolutely stated that the patient was a poor surgical candidate and that surgery would be extremely risky. It does not matter that the patient wanted the surgery. The patient was not an expert on thoracic surgery and surely could not have understood the risks. You were the expert and you exposed the patient to grievous unnecessary risk. You deprived him of several months, perhaps years, of life. You deprived him of the chance to spend his remaining time with his wife, his children, and his grandchildren."

The patient underwent the surgery and the cancer was worse than initially believed. He required not only his left lower lobe to be removed but his entire left lung. Yet he survived and two days later was breathing on his own. Miraculously, the cancer had not spread to his lymph nodes. His breathing would limit strenuous activity but he could again take short walks, travel and spend time with his grandchildren. And he could also hold onto the hope that he was cured of cancer.

In my eyes that surgeon went above and beyond the call of duty and exposed himself to unnecessary liability to save that man's life. What he did was extraordinary yet in his profession ordinary. I shudder when I think of the increasing fear of lawsuits that permeates the surgeon's spirit and prevents him from performing such risky surgeries. I fear that in the near future we will have to watch patients such as this die as we sit by and wonder what happened to the last courageous surgeons.

Refills for Life

The sights and smells of death filled my senses as I entered the room. He was lying on the examining table with his eyes closed. His skin was pale and pasty and his striking weight loss caused his shirt and pants to hang loosely on his body.

"Hi, doctor," his wife brightly greeted me as she stood beside him holding his hand, "he was a little tired and wanted to lie down. Get up dear, the doctor's here."

His eyes flashed open and he gasped for air as he slowly lifted his gaunt frame to a sitting position. I had last seen him one month ago and his deterioration was dramatic. I immediately wondered if I would ever see him again.

"He had his chemo yesterday so he's really tired," his wife explained with a smile, "a couple of more days and he'll be his old self again."

"How are you?" I asked as I shook his hand.

"Hanging in there," he slowly said as he weakly shrugged his shoulders.

He was a seventy year old man who had been my patient for many years. He had suffered a heart attack five years ago but recovered nicely. I treated him for high cholesterol for which he was doing well.

Eighteen months ago he came to me after noticing blood in his urine. He had ignored it at first. He thought it was from aspirin or an infection. When he was finally evaluated he was found to have a large tumor in his right kidney. His kidney was removed but a short time later his cancer was found to have spread to his lungs.

"Did you get his labs back?" his wife asked as he sat passively by her side, "how is his cholesterol?"

His cholesterol had long ago ceased being a serious concern of mine but it remained a concern of hers. There was really no reason to continue treating his cholesterol, as he would likely live only a few more weeks. I felt he should have been in hospice care and our efforts should be towards making him comfortable.

"Real good," I answered, "his cholesterol is very good."

"Did you here that dear," she said, "the doctor said your cholesterol is very good."

He cast his eyes at hers and smiled softly.

We had briefly discussed hospice care at the last visit but she would hear none of it. The oncologist was still treating him with a number of different chemotherapeutic regimens but nothing seemed to be working. But she clung to a determined hope against all reason and would not allow anyone to give up on him.

I examined him and we talked about his overall progress. She explained his latest treatment and tried to convince herself that it would work.

"It's an experimental treatment," she explained, "but his doctor is real excited about it. He says he's heard great things about it. Oh, by the way, he needs a refill on his cholesterol medication."

I pulled out my prescription pad and began writing the prescription.

"Doctor," she added expectantly, "we mail our prescriptions away. Could you make it for ninety days?"

She stared at me with pleading eyes. I knew that there was a real possibility he would not live long enough to receive it in the mail, let alone ninety days. We could both see how he looked. It would only take a thoughtless comment or a hopeless glance to crush her last ray of hope. And that fragile hope was all that sustained her.

I handed her the prescription for the ninety day supply. And I gave her three refills. She smiled appreciatively but I felt a pang of guilt for the emptiness of the gesture. I knew it meant nothing. But to her, it meant everything.

Terri

It was a cold November night as we sat and talked in her cozy second floor sitting room. A Christmas tree cheerfully brightened the room while the TV quietly played in the corner. Cheery get well pictures by neighborhood children hung on the walls. There was an oxygen tank against the wall that allowed her to breathe more comfortably. She was on steady doses of pain medication and held a heating pad tightly against her left chest. I was happy to see her and it was an enjoyable evening.

Her breathing was slightly labored but the conversation was easy. We talked about the office and our years together. We talked about patients who had reached out to her with a card or flowers and how much it meant to her. But just beneath the pleasantness of our conversation tears were quick to surface. She was still reeling from the devastating news of just a few weeks ago. After several months of chemotherapy and dramatic improvement in her symptoms, she was again experiencing pain and shortness of breath. Her cancer was back. There was hopelessness in her eyes.

When we entered our practice we took over file cabinets, examining tables, desks, medical equipment, thousands of wonderful patients, and an excellent staff which included Terri Giorgio. Ten years later, Terri is the only original employee still with us.

Terri has a unique personality that is difficult to describe on paper. She is a robust woman with a loud booming voice. She is never afraid to speak her mind, to tell you the way it is or the way it should be, or to put a person in his place. She can be stubborn, headstrong and proud. If she sounds like a terrible person, nothing could be further from the truth. She somehow pulls off these traits with a disarming, sincere sweetness that causes most people to like her and respect her immediately.

She has held many positions in our practice but primarily does referrals for our HMO patients. The many patients who have dealt with her in their moments of need know how important her role is and how well she does it. Whenever flowers or candy arrive at our office from a patient, we know they are for Terri. She would do whatever was asked, always go that extra mile, never call out sick and always put the interests of our practice and our patients above her own. I have known few people who were so loyal, trustworthy and reliable.

She began having chest pains about six months ago. We immediately feared it was her heart but were even more shattered to learn that she had a small cell cancer in her left lung. We watched her struggle through months of chemotherapy. The intolerable pain, the incessant vomiting, dehydration and severe fatigue. Several times she wanted to give up but somehow persevered.

"I want you to write a story about me," she proudly said as she looked at her CAT scan report a mere two months ago, "I wanted to give up. So many people want to give up. But I stuck it out and now my tumors have all shrunk and I feel great again. I don't know if I can beat this cancer, but I'm going to do everything in my power to fight it."

Terri now finds herself engaged in the battle of her life. In this fight, the cancer seems to have all the advantages. It is an aggressive tumor. It has her lungs, her liver and her bones.

In the ten years that Terri has worked for me, she has quit several times. Something would go wrong and in the heat of the moment she would resign. But her loyalty would force her to give two weeks notice and since she could not stay mad that long she would never actually leave. But more than that, Terri Giorgio is not a quitter.

At fifty-two years of age, there is more that she would like out of life. She has her mother and brother, many relatives and countless friends who are pulling for her.

As we said goodbye that night, she began to talk about the future. She talked about the upcoming holidays and her impending chemotherapy. Beneath the hopelessness in her eyes I saw a fire that burned deeply in her soul. I saw her courage and her toughness. She was ready for the fight.

The cancer may have her lungs, her liver and her bones. But it will never quench her spirit.

Six Days

Six months and six days.

As I paged through his chart for the last time I was intrigued by the time that had passed from his diagnosis until his untimely death. Exactly six months and six days.

It seemed like only yesterday that he was sitting before me, visibly shaken, as we discussed his diagnosis. Yet when I think of all he had went through since that day it seemed more like a hundred years.

"Pancreatic cancer," he said, the shock still fresh on his face, "he said I have pancreatic cancer."

I had seen him one week earlier for abdominal pain and weight loss. He rarely came in to see me so I feared something was seriously wrong. As I examined him, he grimaced when I pressed his left upper abdomen. I had thought that perhaps it was an ulcer but an ultrasound of his abdomen showed a very suspicious mass in his pancreas.

I sent him for a CT scan and had him see a surgeon and an oncologist. I told him what the ultrasound showed but at that point did not have a definitive diagnosis. He was concerned but still optimistic that whatever he had could be treated.

"I read about pancreatic cancer," he continued. "I know it's bad, but I really believe I'm going to beat it. I'm only fifty-seven and I think I'm in great health."

He had seen his oncologist earlier in the day and had received his diagnosis and discussed his treatment options. He was in my office to talk.

"What did he tell you they would do for you?" I asked.

"Well, we didn't get down to specifics," he replied, "but I'm going to see the surgeon tomorrow and probably get chemo. He talked about some experimental treatments that might be an option."

He then looked at the floor and his voiced became tremulous. His blind optimism seemed to be replaced by harsh reality. "He also said that I could do nothing. He said that since I'm not feeling that bad now I could enjoy the time I have left and get hospice care when the time came. He said if I did nothing I would live about six months."

He looked back into my eyes and continued, "Six months. I want to live more than six months. I'm going to do everything in my power to beat this. Everything."

Two days later he had his surgery. The toll it took on his already sick body was devastating. One week later he began chemotherapy.

The treatments he underwent were nearly unbearable yet he persevered. He became so weak that when he was not in the hospital he could rarely leave his house. He could not eat. He could not sleep. The pain was intolerable.

For some, the remarkable treatments that are available for cancer may provide the miracle cure or improve the quality or length of life. For him it gave only a ray of hope, false hope, that he may survive his cancer. Mostly, it just brought more suffering.

Finally, he died alone in a far away hospital while seeking an experimental treatment. His family was notified of his impending death but could not get there in time.

The cost of his treatment approached $200,000, most of which was covered by his insurance company. But the even greater cost could be measured in the blood, pain, and tears that he and his family had paid in full.

As I reflected on his ordeal, I could not help but wonder if perhaps the cost had been too great.

For six days.

15

Heroes

The Fighter

"He was a wonderful man," I said, silently biting my lip in regret for having referred to him in the past tense. "I'll try to get over to see him when I'm through with the patients in my office."

"You mean this afternoon?" the doctor from the intensive care unit asked.

"Yes," I answered, "Why?"

"Well," he slowly replied, "I'm not sure he's going to make it that long."

As I hung up the phone, I was stricken with the realization that his illness was not only worse than I had thought but that he may be dying. He had been a diabetic for years and his wife had called me the night before after having discovered an infected cut on his foot that he was unaware of. He had a fever and seemed confused so I told her to take him to the emergency room.

I finished my morning patients and rushed over to see him during my lunch break. I glanced through his chart and could find little reason for hope. He was in septic shock. His blood gases were terrible despite being on a ventilator. His heart and kidneys were failing. I knew that his underlying condition was poor and that any major insult to his health could put him over the edge. Still, I was surprised with the rapidity of his decline.

He was a delightful and colorful man who had led an incredible life. I had always greatly enjoyed our visits. The history he had seen and participated in during his seventy-six years could fill a book. He had quit high school to join the Marines after Pearl Harbor. He vividly described hitting the beaches of Guadalcanal and watching his beloved American flag flying proudly over the bloodied volcanic soil of Iwo Jima.

His diminutive size was offset by his muscular build and lightning quick hands. While in the Marines, he discovered his true love. Inspired by boxing legend Joe Louis, he began boxing and discovered that he was a natural fighter.

After the war he became a professional boxer and enjoyed some success. While not achieving greatness himself, he had the opportunity to meet and watch the greatest boxers of the time. He vividly described the unforgettable fight in which Rocky Marciano knocked out his hero, Joe Louis. While still a young man, he hung up his gloves forever. He got married, had a family and led a quiet, peaceful life.

In spite of his fascinating stories of the war and professional boxing, his favorite topic was always his grandchildren and the fullness to which he enjoyed his retirement years.

As I stood by his bedside, I sadly realized that the wonderful stories that he so colorfully told would die with him. He was in and out of consciousness, but as I looked into his eyes he was clearly staring back at me. He had a determined look in his eye and I tried my best to hide my despair and convey a look of hope.

He was dying. The cardiologist and nephrologist said so. The chest X-ray and arterial blood gases said so. The kidney function tests said so. But of all the tests performed, there was none that measured the fight in a man's spirit.

And it was the fighter that walked out of the hospital ten days later.

Owen Hart

Step by step he anxiously walked down the long isolated corridor, his eyes fixed on the security guard who led the way.

The few people they passed briefly stared at the young man then quickly looked past him, avoiding any eye contact. Every hair was starkly missing from the young man's head. His severe anemia gave him a ghostly white appearance. His eyes were sunken and his skin hung loosely from his emaciated six-foot frame.

At twenty-six years of age, his future appeared bleak. He was stricken thirteen months prior with a rare and aggressive form of testicular cancer. After two major surgeries and three horrible months of chemotherapy he tried to resume a normal life. But a brief five months later, rising tumor markers and a growth in his right lung indicated that his cancer had returned with a vengeance.

With his life just getting back to normal, he stared blankly as his oncologist explained that he would need to face more surgery and more chemotherapy. At this point, his chance of surviving beyond eighteen months was a mere fifteen percent.

The young man initially approached his latest battle without much hope. He loved to watch a battle, but not when it was he himself who was battling and his life was in the balance. The battles that he most loved to watch took place in a wrestling ring, as he was the great fan of professional wrestling.

The security guard opened a door and led the young man into a small room. Tonight was to be a great night for this professional wrestling fanatic. For tonight in a quiet room of Philadelphia's Spectrum, he was taking a break from his cancer to meet the World Wrestling Federation champion.

The champion humbly entered the room and introduced himself. The two men talked about wrestling and they talked about cancer. As eighteen thousand people awaited his arrival, the champion's full attention was on the young man. The champion offered encouragement as the young man hung on every word. The young patient beamed widely as he tried on the championship belt. The champion introduced his brother, one of professional wrestling's "bad guys", although you never would have known from this meeting.

The two wrestlers were compassionate and gentle. They were inspirational and motivational. No strangers to battle, they respected the great battle the young man was waging. They posed for pictures and signed autographs. They did it not for cameras or publicity, but out of genuine kindness and caring.

Years have passed since that day and of the three men who were there, only two are still living. The young cancer patient fought his battle courageously. Against great odds, he has survived his battle and has enjoyed good health and several more years of Wrestlemania.

The great former champion, Bret Hart, however, lost his brother Owen. The thirty-four year old wrestler, a fine athlete who worked very hard to perfect a difficult art, tragically plunged to his death while entering the ring for a match.

To millions of wrestling fans, Owen Hart will be remembered by his flamboyant bad guy persona. But to at least one young man, he will always be remembered as a caring man whose kindness helped give hope when hope was all but lost.

The Hero

"You're a real lifesaver," she said as she eagerly opened the screen door widely for me. She excitedly extended her arthritic hand towards me and I gingerly grasped it and shook it softly.

"Thank you so much," she continued enthusiastically, "I don't know what we would do without you. It's so hard for me to get him out of bed anymore. It is so nice of you to come out, so thoughtful. Can I get you anything? Would you like something to drink? Here, let me take your coat."

"It really wasn't any trouble," I said as she took my coat and led me down the hall.

The excessiveness of her gratitude made me feel a bit embarrassed yet I knew she meant it sincerely. As I followed her down the narrow hallway I could not help but feel uplifted by her words and proud of what I was doing. After spending the day in my bright and modern medical office, I entered his dark and dated bedroom to provide the care that was so desperately needed.

I had never known him as a healthy man. When I first met him he had already suffered his first stroke which had weakened his left side. He wore a brace over a badly scarred right leg. An "old war injury" he told me, but I never knew the details. He was plagued by further strokes over the next few years. Fortunately they were small strokes, but their cumulative affect had taken their toll. He was also stricken with Parkinson's disease, which had now progressed to an advanced stage. Life would now be confined to his tiny bedroom.

"How are you doing?" I asked as he slowly opened his eyes and looked up at me.

He could not speak but he weakly lifted his trembling arm and I reached down and grasped his hand. He was a small man, probably not more than five feet, five inches tall and I doubt that he even weighed a hundred pounds. He looked so tiny and frail in his oversized hospital bed.

I carefully examined him then asked his wife if she had something with which I could clean a large bedsore. She excused herself and slowly walked out of the room.

I stood alone for what seemed an eternity. My eyes wandered the room. Old paintings and family photographs covered the walls. I stepped towards their dresser and smiled as I examined them as a young couple in their wedding picture, she as a beautiful young woman in her wedding dress and he as a handsome young man smiling smartly in his army uniform.

Towards the back of the dresser there was an inconspicuously placed old military decoration. His wife had still not returned so I bent over to read the citation.

"Normandy, France, 23 June 1944: For conspicuous gallantry and intrepidity at risk of life above and beyond the call of duty, for twice exposing himself to withering enemy machinegun and mortar fire to reach and carry to safety two seriously wounded comrades. His dauntless courage was entirely responsible for saving the two soldiers' lives."

I stood humbly by his bed and stared in disbelief at the frail little man. I no longer saw a pitiful, helpless patient. I looked beyond the oversized hospital bed and the side rails, the paralyzed body and muted voice, the catheters, diapers, and broken down skin. And there lie a hero.

Dr. Francesconi

I remember the first time I met him. It was my third year of medical school and I had just spent time working with a family doctor. I had always wanted to be a family doctor and had looked forward to the experience.

The doctor I had worked with had an excellent reputation, a take charge personality and sharp clinical skills. His patients hated him. He always seemed rushed, agitated and never quite at ease with them. I often wonder why patients stay with doctors they don't like. But they do.

It was an unpleasant experience and I had begun to doubt my career choice as I began my full family practice rotation. I entered the office and timidly introduced myself to the receptionist. Before she could answer, the doctor came bounding from his office.

"Al Francesconi," he said as he excitedly shook my hand, "it's a pleasure to meet you. You're going to love this rotation. We'll have a good time together. You're going to learn a lot."

I was taken by surprise at his enthusiastic reception. As a medical student I had never been treated this way by an attending physician. In the medical hierarchy, a medical student is valued far below an intern and slightly above a bedpan. He treated me like a colleague, an equal, a long lost friend.

He was short in stature but big in heart. He loved to teach and always had a story to tell. His patients liked him. No, his patients loved him. He taught me a great deal about treating illnesses. But more importantly, he taught me about treating people. It was during those weeks that I firmly made up my mind to become a family doctor.

We kept in touch through the years. He provided valuable guidance to me as I established my own practice. We talked about our lives, medicine, and the health problems that began to plague his life. He had a condition called non-alcoholic steatohepatitis. This basically meant that through no fault of his own his liver was slowly failing. Eventually he would need a liver transplant.

In June of 2001, he merged his practice with ours in anticipation of his eventual transplant. It was exciting to again work with him but his illness had taken its toll. After a long and agonizing wait, he received his liver in November, 2002. For a while he was his old self again. He had a bounce in his step, more stories to tell, and excitedly returned to his profession. Unfortunately, within six months his new liver was failing.

He continued to work as his doctors struggled to help him. When his doctors and family advised him to quit working he argued that his patients were his best therapy. As I look back, I am astonished that he was able to continue working as long as he did. He never complained and I doubt that his patients were aware that it was shear courage and mental determination that allowed him to drag himself through the workday. He could no longer even write his notes yet still would not abandon his profession.

I'll never forget the last time I saw him. He finally admitted that he could no longer work and asked me if I would take over with his medical student.

"This is the last student scheduled until January," he said, then added, "if I'm still alive."

"Don't say that," his student said, "you'll be alive."

He just shrugged. He knew. That's the problem with being a doctor. You know.

I told him that I would cover for him. If I had known it would be the last time I would ever see him I would have said more. In my mind I may have known he was dying but in my heart I did not believe it.

Over the next week he suffered a GI bleed, his kidneys shut down, he developed peritonitis and respiratory failure. After talking to his wife on July 28, a mere seven days after his last day of work, for the first time I realized that he was going to die. He died a few hours later.

I could fill several pages with stories of Dr. Francesconi as a husband, a father, a loyal friend and a Vietnam veteran. But I knew him as a doctor. He was the only man that I ever considered a mentor. And probably ever will be.

Many of his patients are now my patients. Every day I listen to their stories of the great Dr. Francesconi. Teary-eyed stories of a down to earth man who touched so many lives and who will be so sorely missed.

I will always consider myself privileged to have been among his students. And like the many students before and after me, I know that Dr. Albert Francesconi will be a part of me always.

Boyhood Hero

I looked at his name on my schedule. I wanted to see him. I really did. But I no longer looked forward to seeing him. Absent was the pleasant banter about sports, his vacations and his family that used to mark our visits. He was in the final stages of bone cancer. He had valiantly fought his fight but unfortunately after three years seemed to be losing. He was no longer being treated aggressively. He had chronic pain, but otherwise his physical quality of life was not bad. Emotionally, however, he was becoming increasingly despondent. I could listen to him, but there was little I could do to help him.

I knocked on the examining room door and slowly opened it. I had last seen him a month ago and was unsure how much he may have deteriorated.

"Good morning," I cautiously offered.

"Good morning, Doc," he enthusiastically replied, his smile lighting up the room.

"So, how are you doing?" I expectantly inquired.

His smile dimmed but slightly. He was a diminutive seventy-two year old man, barely five foot six inches tall, with thinning gray hair and a pale complexion.

"Uh, not much better," he answered, "I guess about the same."

I wondered what had caused the dramatic change in his outlook but knew I wouldn't have to wait long to find out.

"I didn't know John was your patient," he said, referring to the next patient on my schedule, "I've been coming here for ten years and never saw him before. Didn't even know he lived near here. Boy, does that take me back. I'll bet I haven't seen John in thirty . . . thirty-five years. We used to work together at the shipyard. I was a tool maker then, the supervisor in the shop and John was an apprentice. He was a good kid . . . a big kid . . . he used to play baseball, semi-pro I think."

John was no longer a kid. He was still a very big, friendly man but he was in his early sixties, suffered from diabetes and had undergone coronary artery bypass surgery three years earlier. It was nice for these old acquaintances to meet but I still didn't understand the complete transformation.

"Interesting story about John and I," he excitedly explained, "I remember when John started and I barely knew him. It was a payday and I had cashed my check and was walking out to my car late one night. It was real dark. All of a sudden these two thugs came out of nowhere and demanded my money. One of them shoved me against my car and started punching me. I was stupid. I should have just given them the money. But we had just had a baby and I really needed the money. 'Give me your money or we'll kill you,' they shouted. They knocked me hard to the ground. Started kicking me."

I could see the fear in his eyes as he vividly recounted the frightening memory.

"I just held on to my wallet and braced myself," he continued, "then I heard this horrible crash. I thought I was a dead man but then I realized they didn't hit me. I looked up and saw the one guy flying across the hood of my car. Then someone punched the other guy and he went crashing to the ground."

Tears filled his eyes but his face could not stop smiling.

"It was John," he said, "the kid saved my life."

A strange and wonderful coincidence had led him to his friend after all those many years. He left that day a contented man and died a few weeks later. I don't know if he had any dying wishes. But I will never forget the joy on his face that day and always remember how much it means to a dying man to meet his boyhood hero.

Sergeant Schmidt

September meant reunion time. As the years passed, every fall brought more and more significance to William W. Schmidt and his buddies from the 36th Cavalry Recon Tank Squadron. They all shared a common bond, World War II veterans that had fought and survived through battles in France, Belgium and Germany.

Bill Schmidt had been my patient since my residency. He was a big and tough man with weathered skin and a gravelly voice. When you first meet him he may come across as gruff but it only takes a few moments to appreciate his warmth and down-to-earth manner. He had a no-nonsense, get-things-done way about him that must have served him well as a sergeant in the army, at his job at the electric company, and as a Commander of his American Legion Post. But I never saw him as anything short of a gentleman. He was a caring human being and a devoted family man. He had been married for fifty-seven years to his lovely wife Audrey and cherished his children and his grandchildren.

I would see him frequently over the many years that he was my patient and we had forged a close bond. At seventy-nine years of age, he continued to radiate the appearance of strength and of confidence. But just beneath his apparent vigor were many serious medical problems. The only visible evidence was his need for the use of a cane, the result of a stroke that had left him weakened. But he also suffered from emphysema, high blood pressure, high cholesterol, prostate and colon cancer that had spread to his liver.

Every summer he would see all of his specialists in preparation for the fall journey. I would usually see him just before he left. There were times that I worried if he was in good enough shape to make the trip but it was impossible to stand in the way of his enthusiasm. In all the years that I had known him, he had only missed one reunion and that was following major surgery for his colon cancer.

When he returned from his trip, he would come in to see me and we would discuss any problems that he may have had. Uplifted by the support of his lifelong friends, he never had any serious trouble. Most of the office visit would be spent listening to the stories of his trip, tales of tourists exploring diverse areas of the country and of old soldiers sharing war stories. I sat in awe as he would humbly recount his wartime experiences. I remember a few years back when he played host and everyone came to New Jersey. He enthusiastically spoke of the planning, the meetings, and the camaraderie. He was in his glory as host to all of his friends.

Last year he traveled to Portland, Oregon, to a reunion hosted by his friend Earl Carpenter. Amidst the joy of the reunion, there was the sadness of the friends that were no longer there. Friends like Keith Wanderlich from Iowa who had lost his battle against cancer and Ray Guilliland of Colorado who had succumbed to emphysema. They had diseases that Bill Schmidt shared.

As the years passed, his health became more fragile. He continued to convey a certain vigor about him but I knew that the slightest disturbance could spell disaster. It came in the form of an innocuous bleeding sore on his nose. He went to the hospital where a biopsy of the bleeding site revealed skin cancer. It seemed like a minor problem and the plastic surgeon routinely removed the cancer. But shortly thereafter he suffered a stroke and died a few days later.

When John Brewer hosts this year's reunion in New Orleans on September 15, William W. Schmidt will be among the missing. He will join his friends who have died over the years. He will also join the men who have never had the opportunity to attend a reunion. Men like Howard Alber, felled by a sniper's bullet in Normandy, France. Men like Gerard Krug and Robert Heddelson who were cut down by machine gun fire near the Ruhr River in Germany. Men like Sherrod Simpson who was killed by mortar fire and Warren Sams who was killed by an artillery shell. Brave men who gave their last full measure of devotion to their country.

On a warm summer's evening as I silently walked from the funeral home, I realized how much I would miss Bill Schmidt and his wonderful talent for bringing history to life.

Rest in peace Sergeant Schmidt, and may you enjoy the reunion.

16

Goodbye

Farewell to a Friend

I quickly parked my car and walked hurriedly towards the door. To my regret, the service had already started so I quietly found a seat towards the back of the crowded chapel.

Except for the sound of weeping, there was only a respectful silence as her rabbi described the full and wonderful life of a teacher, wife, mother, daughter and friend that had ended too soon at the age of fifty-three.

I don't remember the first time I met her. Her routine complaint at that time has long ago escaped my memory. Over the years, our patient-doctor relationship developed with each visit. She was a delightful woman and our conversations would often slip well beyond her scheduled appointment.

Two and a half years ago she presented to me with a firm, enlarging lump in her neck. I breathed deeply as I silently palpated the suspicious mass. She could read the concern on my face as I told her she would need to have a biopsy performed.

Non-Hodgkin's lymphoma. A low-grade malignancy she was told. She should live a normal life. These words would haunt her as her disease shadowed her every move.

Every course of chemotherapy seemed to bring a response, perhaps a cure. But then there it was again, another lymph node or an abnormal X-ray proving that her cancer was relentlessly stalking her.

I saw her frequently throughout her ordeal. We talked about her physical and emotional struggles, her hopes and her fears. But we also talked about more everyday matters such as our jobs and our families.

Her strength and courage never failed to astound me. During her chemotherapy, she often looked so sick that I wondered why she was not in the hospital. Then she would tell me that that very day she was in school teaching.

Somewhere deep in our hearts and minds, most doctors draw a line of emotional detachment. It allows us to treat our patients objectively. It lets us share a tear with a dying patient and then ten minutes later laugh at the antics of a healthy two year old. We can comfort a young mother who has lost a child, then go home and play with our own children. It allows us to sleep at night.

But with each tearful embrace at the end of every emotional visit, I knew that line had long ago been crossed.

I will never forget the last time I saw her. She had a draining incision and needed to see a surgeon. I asked my receptionist to make the arrangements while I saw my next patient. The surgeon asked her to come right over. When I returned, she was gone. It seemed like a routine problem and I did not know at the time that I would never see her again. I never got to say goodbye.

She taught school on a Wednesday and celebrated Thanksgiving with her family on Thursday. She died on Saturday.

I felt strongly compelled to attend her funeral. I sensed a need to offer my condolences to her family or perhaps I felt it was my final duty as her doctor. But as I sat silently in my chair and tears welled in my eyes, I realized that more than anything else I had come for myself. I needed to say goodbye to a friend.

Buerger's Disease

"Man, they tell me I got some hamburger disease," he said with a hearty laugh, "I guess I've been eating too much McDonald's and it clogged my veins."

I curiously looked through his chart as his stretcher was parked in the radiology department's hallway. As an intern, it had been my job to accompany this ICU patient during his transport.

"Buerger's disease," I said as I shared in his laughter.

"That's what I said," he replied, "eating too much hamburgers."

I had never seen a case of Buerger's disease and remembered little about it. "It's not about hamburgers," I explained, "I think it's about cigarettes."

"You got some cigarettes," he playfully asked, "I haven't had one in two days."

"No," I smiled, "Buerger's disease is something you can see in smokers. I think it causes the arteries of the legs and arms to close off."

I was not sure of the facts, but he didn't know any better. He looked at me curiously then looked at his right hand.

"That why my fingertips are blue?" he asked as he showed me his cold and blue right index and middle finger.

He was a thin, pleasant young black man. He told me he was from Chicago but I don't remember why he had left. He seemed healthy but for this one problem. We sat there together joking and laughing for a long time. I was not permitted to leave so I relaxed and tried to enjoy my wait. After half an hour, he seemed to become confused and agitated. He tried to climb out of his bed and became combative. At first I tried to calm him down by friendly words but quickly realized he did not comprehend. He swung wildly at me. I grabbed his arms and leaned my weight against his chest. I called for help. I wasn't laughing anymore.

"He had a couple of friends visit him a little while ago," a muscular ER technician reported as he roughly tied down the young man's arms, "I'll bet they gave him drugs."

The young man did have a past history of drug abuse and the offhand comment quickly became the working diagnosis: Buerger's disease and a drug overdose.

Two days later, my curiosity led me to a private room at the end of a hall. He lay unconscious, kept alive by a ventilator. I perused his chart to see what had happened to him. There was no longer any mention of Buerger's disease or a drug overdose. He had damaged heart valves and a blood clot in his heart. He was throwing clots throughout his body. They had occluded the arteries of his hand and showered the circulation of his brain. He was brain dead. Unable to contact any family members, the hospital ethics committee had decided to discontinue life support.

I sat in his room as the respiratory technician came in to pull the plug. I thought the scene would be more memorable, but he simply turned the machine off. I thought it would be quick, but it was excruciatingly slow. Deprived of oxygen, his heart began racing before gradually slowing down and becoming irregular. I scanned the room. The only personal effects were two strange looking greeting cards with pictures of flowers and Japanese tapestries and affectionate "thinking of you" words. They were both signed "with love" by the same woman. I wondered who she was. I wondered where she was.

The respiratory technician left the room. I sat down beside the young man and stared at his fading heart monitor. It seemed so terribly sad that he would die so utterly alone in a strange place. I got up to leave but realized that I was the last person there, the last person he had talked to, and the closest thing he had to a friend. I sat back down and squeezed his hand and silently watched his heartbeat fade away.

Saying Goodbye

He stood up as I entered the room and had an uncomfortable look on his face as if he had something he needed to tell me.

"Good morning," I said as I extended my hand towards him.

"Good morning, doctor," he replied as he held onto my hand a little longer than usual.

He was a seventy-five year old retired city policeman. I saw him frequently since his bypass surgery five years ago and aggressively treated his high blood pressure and high cholesterol. He was diagnosed with prostate cancer three years ago but it had progressed very slowly and he was being treated conservatively.

To look at him, he was the picture of good health. He looked fit and trim with thick gray hair, broad shoulders and a ready smile. His mind was sharp as a tack and he could have passed for ten years younger. He still conveyed a feeling of strength. Even with his advancing age, you felt safe in his presence.

Our visit progressed as usual. I asked how he was doing and if he had any problems. I examined him and reviewed his lab work. Everything seemed to be going well.

Although he saw me regularly, he and his wife would travel to Southern California for months at a time to visit his son's family. As the years passed, he frequently talked about one day moving out to be near the only family he had.

"Have you been out to see your son lately?" I asked.

"Yes, as a matter of fact I was there last month," he answered.

"Are you still planning on moving there permanently someday?" I asked.

"Actually, I think this will be the last time you'll be seeing me," he answered, his voice cracking, "we just sold our house and we're moving next month."

I could tell that he was upset to have to tell me the news. It is always hard to say goodbye, but he was not dying or going into a nursing home. This should have been a happy goodbye. Still, after all of these years I knew I would never see him again.

As the visit ended I took his hand into both of mine.

"It's been a great pleasure to have you as a patient all these years," I told him reassuringly. "I always hate to lose such nice patients but I'm very happy for you. If there is anything I can do for you just let me know."

As I held his right hand in mine, he reached out with his left hand then pulled it abruptly to his face. I didn't see it coming and I know that he didn't either. Tears started streaming down his face and he struggled to stop their flow and regain his composure. I was touched by his emotions and felt tears welling in my own eyes.

"Thank you doctor," he said through the tears, "I'll miss you too."

He smiled weakly as he wiped his eyes then walked slowly from the office.

You never realize how deeply you may touch a patient's life. I watched him walk out of the office that day and never saw him again. He could have written me a card or sent candy or flowers to thank me for what I had done. But instead he broke down and cried. I could not have received a more heartfelt gift.

The Greatest Lesson

I knocked on the door and entered the room. Most of the furniture had been removed to make room for a large hospital bed that contained a frail elderly woman. A lone lamp cast a haunting shadow across her face. She turned slowly towards me as I approached.

"How are you?" I asked.

She smiled weakly and whispered a faint, "okay."

She was in the final stages of ovarian cancer. She had been through the surgeries and the chemotherapy. She had seen all of the specialists. She had gotten second opinions and third opinions but the answers were always the same. She had failed all the treatments they had tried and there was nothing more they could do. She was now in hospice care. Her treatment would now be directed towards making her comfortable in her dwindling final days.

Her walls were lined with kindergarten class pictures. Every one of them with her as a petite and gently aging schoolteacher smiling proudly with her arms around her brightly beaming students.

She was as prepared as a person could be for the ordeal she was facing. She was spiritually ready to die. Still, she was understandably frightened. Tears welled in her eyes and rolled down her cheek. I held her hand and stroked her face to wipe away the tears.

I stared at her face. In my mind she was transfigured to the prime of her life. I could envision her liveliness and her voice as she lifted the hearts and minds of scores of children with stories and songs, laughter and love. But that time of innocence was long over. Her beautiful voice would soon be silent.

I looked into her eyes. Despite her illness and her age, her eyes remained as blue as the sky. In her eyes I saw my own kindergarten teacher and long forgotten memories stirred within me. I remembered holding my mother's hand as she led me to my first day of school. I stood there bravely as my mother kissed me goodbye then walked down the hall leaving me alone for the first time in a strange place. I stood by the door, frozen with fear as tears began filling my eyes.

An angel approached. It was my kindergarten teacher. She smiled and wiped away my tears. She held my hand and asked me my name. She lovingly led me to my classroom to begin my formal education that would span more than twenty years and conclude with a degree in medicine.

In the faces of the children in the pictures I saw myself. I was thankful for my teacher and in the same way felt a debt of gratitude towards my dying patient. All of the years of education. All of the teachers. All of the studying. My gratitude transformed to the frustrating realization that despite all I had been taught over all those years, I had not learned anything that could now help my dying patient.

Tears welled in my eyes as I looked back into her face. As I held her hand, she smiled softly and a peacefulness seemed to replace her fear. A smile came over my face. In all of my years of schooling, there was only one thing I had ever learned that could help her. And that was the love and kindness taught me by my own kindergarten teacher on my first day of school nearly forty years ago.